WOMEN IN MEDICINE

This book is dedicated to the hundreds of women physicians and medical students who have shared their experiences and stories with me over the years—the primary sources of my medical education.

JANET BICKEL

WOMEN IN MEDICINE

Getting In, Growing, and Advancing

Sage Publications, Inc.
International Educational and Professional Publisher
Thousand Oaks ■ London ■ New Delhi

For information:

Sage Publications, Inc.
2455 Teller Road
Thousand Oaks, California 91320
E-mail: order@sagepub.com

Sage Publications Ltd.
6 Bonhill Street
London EC2A 4PU
United Kingdom

Sage Publications India Pvt. Ltd.
M-32 Market
Greater Kailash I
New Delhi 110 048 India

Printed in the United States of America

Library of Congress Cataloging-in-Publication Data

Bickel, Janet W.
  Women in medicine: Getting in, growing, and advancing / by Janet
Bickel.
      p. cm. — (Surviving medical school ; v. 4)
  Includes bibliographical references and index.
    ISBN 0-7619-1818-3 (cloth: acid-free paper)
    ISBN 0-7619-1819-1 (pbk: acid-free paper)
    1. Women in medicine. 2. Women medical students. I. Title. II.
Series.
    R692 .B498 2000
    610'.82—dc21

                                99-050605

This book is printed on acid-free paper.

00   01   02   03   04   05   06   7   6   5   4   3   2   1

Acquisition Editor:	Rolf Janke
Editorial Assistant:	Heidi Van Middlesworth
Production Editor:	Sanford Robinson
Editorial Assistant:	Cindy Bear
Typesetter:	Tina Hill
Indexer:	Molly Hall
Cover Designer:	Candice Harman

Contents

Foreword

Women physicians, increasing in number, are enjoying the challenges and rewards of their profession. However, they still encounter barriers to the achievement of their professional and personal goals, some societal and common to all professional women, and others unique to medicine.

Janet Bickel, America's best-informed scholar on this topic, has written this insightful book culled from decades of teaching and research with women in medicine. An empathetic, insightful, and practical approach in this "must-read" primer, they discuss the unique problems these women face and the personal and professional skills needed to succeed in medicine today.

Janet Bickel, M.S., Associate Vice President of the Association of American Medical Colleges (AAMC), has worked at the forefront of medical education for over 25 years. Most recently she has focused on planning and development in medical education, keying in on issues related to women. A renowned speaker at national meetings and more than sixty-five medical centers, Ms. Bickel publishes articles on a broad spectrum of areas in academic medicine, including students' and residents' ethical development. She also directs the AAMC's Women in Medicine program, where she has developed and implemented a series of professional development seminars for women leaders in academic medicine. These have received excellent reviews from more than 2,000 faculty members who have attended.

As more and more women enter medicine—currently 43% of medical school classes are female—the dynamics of this profession will continue to change dramatically. As such, men as well as women would be wise to peruse the valuable contents of this book.

—Robert Holman Coombs
Professor of Biobehavioral Sciences, UCLA School of Medicine
Series Editor

Acknowledgments

The author thanks Renee Marshall Lawson for her superb and patient administrative assistance throughout this project and also Kathy M. Croft for her research and editorial assistance.

Introduction

What is unsought will go undetected.
—*Sophocles*

No wonder so many women are choosing to become physicians. Medicine offers abundant and diverse opportunities to take care of individuals, improve public health, advance science, make a good living, and become a leader in the community, in an academic center, and in professional organizations. To be sure, the choice to pursue medicine is not an easy one; it is a big investment, and not every young woman's family will be supportive. But if you have a solid academic record and the determination, you can become a great physician.

The demand for women physicians just keeps growing as more and more women health care consumers actively and specifically seek them—and not just for birth control advice and Pap smears. If offered a choice, many women would also prefer a woman breast surgeon, pediatrician, dermatologist, and psychiatrist. The power of women as health care consumers is just beginning to be recognized. Women make three fourths of the health care decisions in American households and spend almost two of three health care dollars.

This is also an exciting time in history relative to women's health. The complexities of women's life cycles and the largest causes of mortality in women—for instance, heart disease and breast cancer—have only recently begun to receive hefty research funding and the attention of medical educators, public policy makers, and physicians across the board.

Women no longer feel like newcomers to medicine. They now make up 43% of entering classes in medical schools, up from 5% 50 years ago. With all this progress, some women and men might legitimately question the need for a book targeted at women. They might similarly question the value of women's groups or meetings. If invited to an open house sponsored by the women faculty organization, some women medical students might ask "What are those old fogies still talking about?" and some men might respond "Is this a plot against the men here?"

As a glance at this book's table of contents reveals, there is still a lot to talk about. Gender inequality is still characteristic of our culture, with men's careers more highly valued than women's, and the medical profession is not immune from these cultural inequities. So compared with men, women in medicine still face extra challenges in the development and valuing of their skills and potential.

However, none of the issues dealt with here are "women's issues"; they are societal issues, the responsibility and concern of men and women both. Improvements to ensure that women have equal access to all career options and resources will not only enhance what women can contribute to the profession but will ultimately improve the quality of patient care and research in this country.

The primary aim of this book is to help women entering medicine to maximize their options and to have the fullest possible lives and careers. Actually, because men and women share so many characteristics and needs, much of the research cited and advice contained here is relevant to both. But building as it does on all the best available literature and studies on gender differences and on the experience of thousands of women physicians who have come before you, this book is designed for women. An added benefit is that all but the last chapter conclude with a "Diagnose Yourself" section, to help you personalize the content, to stimulate you to begin necessary preparations, and to support you along the journey.

Most chapters are relevant for anyone considering a medical career whether they be in junior high school or in their 40s and contemplating a major life change. In this regard, it will also be of interest to health professions advisers and to teachers who want to be better mentors to students considering becoming a physician. Medical students and young physicians in residency training will also find here a great deal of practical guidance. The book is also a resource that can be referred to again later—for instance, when it comes time to interview for a job.

A couple of disclaimers. First, women are just as different from each other as men are from each other, so any generalization here about women will certainly not hold true for all women. Moreover, the special issues facing ethnic minorities, disabled women, and lesbians are barely touched on. However, the Association of American Medical Colleges' (AAMC) *Medical School Admission Requirements* (Varner, 1999; see Chapter 1) does include sections addressed to minority applicants and to disabled students. Lesbians can get advice before and after medical school entry from the American Medical Student Association's (AMSA) Lesbian, Gay & Bisexual People in Medicine Task Force and from the Gay and Lesbian Medical Association (see Appendix F).

One piece of advice is offered up front: Most women entering medicine want to "have it all"—a thriving practice, academic pursuits, a loving partner, healthy children, plus personal time! But no one can have it all, all at once. Understanding what is ahead and evaluating your options at every stage will mean wiser choices and prioritizing. That is how to maximize the resilience of your career and the satisfaction you find overall.

1 Getting Into the Medical School and Residency You Want

> Beginnings are apt to be shadowy.
> —*Rachel Carson*

So you have decided on a career in medicine. Now how do you get a corner on the medical school admissions process? How competitive do you have to be? How do medical schools assess motivation? How do you find the medical school that is the best match for you? You will find succinct advice in the first section of this chapter, which concludes with advice for nontraditional applicants.

The second section of this chapter is a realistic look at why women students have continuing concerns about equity and offers an orientation to what women can expect once they begin medical school. This section may also give you ideas about areas to explore during medical school interviews.

After starting medical school, the next major decision is deciding on a specialty and a residency training program. Women often need encouragement to consider the full range of possibilities, including surgery and biomedical research. Therefore, this section gets you started thinking early and broadly about your options. The last sections will help you prepare for your interviews for both medical school and residency.

1

First Things First:
Becoming Competitive and Selecting a School

For the last several years, women have demonstrated a slight edge over men in gaining acceptance to medical school. For instance, in the class admitted in the 1998 to 1999 academic year, 41.7% of men applicants were accepted compared with 43.2% of women. Because women tend overall to score lower than men on the Medical College Admission Test (MCAT) and to present a lower science grade point average (GPA), in general they must be stronger in the other areas that schools most value. As an aside, of women gaining admission to medical school, women's colleges produce almost twice as high a proportion as any other category of undergraduate preparation (Tidball, Smith, Tidball, & Wolf-Wendell, 1998). Clearly, a favorable climate for women students is one where they see many women role models seriously engaged in a variety of academic pursuits.

Just what are medical schools looking for? Medical schools review candidates with special attention to the following areas: personal qualities, academic qualifications, communication skills, and motivation. Naturally, most schools are looking for the most highly academically qualified students they can attract. To give you an idea of what it takes to be competitive with regard to academic qualifications, in 1998, 80% of matriculants had undergraduate GPAs of 3.26 or higher. The majority of accepted applicants with lower GPAs achieved relatively high scores on the MCAT; only 5% of accepted applicants had GPAs lower than 3.0. In addition to these signs of academic determination, medical schools also look for certain science prerequisites, especially physics and chemistry.

Motivation is perhaps the most salient nonintellectual trait sought by most admission committees. A competitive medical school applicant will have not only a general understanding of the profession but also a demonstrated interest in and knowledge of what the field of medicine encompasses. You can demonstrate your interest and deepen your knowledge by working in health care settings (paid or volunteer, especially in a clinical setting), talking with health professionals, reading current literature about medicine and health, and doing research at the undergraduate level. In addition to evidence of maturity, all medical schools are also seeking evidence of commitment to lifelong learning and to serving the public. The research-oriented schools are especially seeking students who are turned on by laboratory and clinical research and who may become clinical investigators (Heinig, Quon, Meyer, & Korn, 1999).

The best source of specifics on each school's prerequisites and characteristics is the Association of American Medical College's (AAMC; see Appendix F) annual guide, *Medical School Admission Requirements (MSAR)* (Varner, 1999). It describes all accredited medical schools in the United States and Canada. Another useful resource is AAMC's annual *Curriculum Directory* which describes the academic programs, required courses, and educational innovations. The AAMC Publications Office is planning a supplemental CD-ROM companion for the 2000 to 2001 edition. AAMC offers MSAR_ Clipboard, an electronic mailing list for students and applicants with news about application deadlines, admission policies and procedures, test dates, AAMC-sponsored Career Awareness Workshops, and other publications for medical students.

For applicants still in college, the most valuable resource of all for premedical planning and advice on school selection is the undergraduate prehealth adviser. The earlier you introduce yourself to this person the better, even if you are still not sure you want to apply to medical school, because this person can help you consider all your options.

Once you have done your basic research on the lay of land and have some feel for where you would like to be and where you have some chance of acceptance, you can start looking in more depth for a match between your interests and characteristics and those of the schools. For most students, state of residency, tuition, and financial aid availability are the most important variables (again, *MSAR* is your best starting point on these issues). Another consideration for some is where your friends live or may be going.

Naturally many women applicants would prefer a school with a long track record of attracting and accepting women students. Included in *MSAR* is a table showing the numbers and proportions of women applicants, new entrants, and total enrollees at each school. In the 1998 to 1999 academic year, women made up the majority of new entrants at 21 of the 125 schools. The Uniformed Services University had the lowest proportion of women new entrants (22%) and University of Missouri-Columbia (61%) the highest. The "low" and the "high" school are usually different each year.

Naturally, many women applicants would prefer a school with a lot of women on faculty and in leadership positions and an appropriate portion of the curricula devoted to women's health issues. Also preferable is an environment where women's needs and careers are taken as seriously as men's. Another feature of interest is campus safety and security. No "all purpose" data source exists on these scores; you have to do some digging.

AAMC's annual *Women in U.S. Academic Medicine Statistics* (Bickel, Croft, & Marshall, 1998) provides a national status report on women applicants, students, residents, faculty, and administrators (see Appendices B and F). Also included for the first time in 1997 are results from AAMC's new annual Benchmarking Survey designed to determine the extent of women's leadership and advancement at U.S. medical schools. This publication now displays, for virtually all U.S. medical schools, the proportion of women faculty and professors and the numbers of women division chiefs, department chairs, and deans. For each school the number of women on institutional committees and the amount of funding to support programming for women are shown. Although these indices are not a measure of equity per se, a comparatively low proportion of women faculty should raise some questions in your mind, and the additional profiled information can provide insight into the school's gender climate.

Next, check out *Enhancing the Environment for Women in Academic Medicine: Resources and Pathways* (Bickel, Croft, & Marshall, 1996), a resource guide downloadable from the AAMC Website (see Appendix F). This book contains numerous examples from schools across the country of recent work and improvements of interest to women. An example along these lines from the University of Virginia School of Medicine is a Gender Fairness Environment Scale, a useful tool developed by their Committee on Women (see Appendix C).

With regard to finding a "gender issues perspective" in the clinical curricula, look for acknowledgment that women and men have different life experiences, risk factors, and present health problems differently (for more on women's health, see Chapter 6). Also look for recognition of the impact of violence in intimate relationships, respect of cultural diversity and sexual orientation, and gender-neutral language in publications and lectures (Lent & Bishop, 1998).

Naturally, if you have a young child (or are hoping to soon have one), you will also be alert to whether the medical center has on-site day care. Ask about the length of the waiting list, about the cost (and whether any financial support is possible), and about day care alternatives in the community.

A possible resource on some of these school characteristics is the local American Medical Women's Association (AMWA) chapter. Although not all locales have an active AMWA chapter, where there is one, you can get help with a large variety of questions, especially relative to gender climate. Some chapters may offer help with housing while you are there for an interview. When there is no AMWA chapter, ask the school's admissions office for the names of local women physicians who might be willing to answer questions about the school and visit the AMWA's Website (see Appendix F).

Bottom line: An excellent medical education can be obtained at any U.S. medical school. But take a practical approach in your search with regard to location and financing. If you have the opportunity, seek a school where gender equity is highly valued. The most critical ingredients, however, in your acquiring a solid medical education are your own initiative and commitment to learning.

Considerations for the Nontraditional Student

Nontraditional to most medical schools equals "out of college," and the above applies most directly to students applying to medical school directly from or shortly after college. What about those coming to medicine from another career or after a number of years caring for a family? It is no longer uncommon for registered nurses and a wide array of other health professionals to outgrow their first careers and seek the decision-making capability the medical degree provides. The numbers of older applicants have increased slightly in recent years, such that now about 5% of accepted applicants are more than 32 years old. However, as shown in *MSAR*, the acceptance rate tends to decrease with age; whereas 52% of applicants age 21 to 23 achieve acceptance, only 25% of applicants age 35 to 37 do.

These lower acceptance rates are largely a result of lower GPAs and MCAT scores; also admissions committees may have doubts about how "fresh" the individual's study skills and science prerequisites are. Some students therefore return to school (often while continuing other responsibilities) to retake key medical school prerequisites. An even more serious alternative is to enter a structured "postbaccalaureate" program designed for applicants to medical school (see *MSAR* for details).

The upside for "mature" applicants, especially those coming from the health field, is that admissions committees often find it easier to assess their motivation. With their higher levels of self-knowledge, responsibility and adaptive strategies, older applicants tend to be "safer bets" than less mature college students.

Differences Between
Men and Women Medical Students

Why do some women students have continuing concerns about equity in medical education? What should you be prepared to deal with? And are the career plans and perspectives that men and women bring to medical school more alike than different? The following section is a "heads up" from recent research on medical students.

Each year the AAMC surveys all students matriculating into a U.S. medical school. For the most part, women and men matriculants look more alike than different. One interesting area of difference that endures from year to year is that, compared with men, women give higher emphasis to community service, patient education, and psychological aspects of patient care; medical schools are increasingly looking for these values so it is not surprising that a higher proportion of women than men are accepted. Men tend to give greater weight than women to high professional achievement, high income prospects, and high status and prestige (Bickel & Ruffin, 1994). Similar gender differences in career-related values are evident from surveys of high school students.

AAMC also surveys all students graduating from U.S. medical schools. A higher proportion of women than men rate curricular coverage of numerous subjects as inadequate, especially family and domestic violence, medical care cost control, and public health (Bickel & Ruffin, 1994). It could be that women's expectations of curricular coverage are higher than men's. Alternatively, with men comprising three quarters of medical school faculty, some of whom may be more comfortable with men than women trainees, it is possible that the quality of women's education is not up to par with men's. One study of a surgery clerkship, for example, found that women's performance was equivalent to men's, but the women gave lower ratings than men to 12 of 15 aspects of the clerkship, including attitudes of the staff and skill development opportunities (Calkins, Willoughby, & Arnold, 1992). Another educational deficit pointed out by women is that some medical textbooks still depict the male body as "the norm," thus physicians are likely not developing as complete a knowledge of normal female anatomy (Mendelsohn, Nieman, Isaacs, Lee, & Levison, 1994).

Although most medical schools are working to correct such deficiencies in their formal curricula, some aspects of the "informal" curriculum are harder to address—for instance, the pressures on medical students and physicians to cultivate detachment and indifference (Bickel, 1994). A study of first-year medical students' reactions to human dissection and to terminally ill patients found that women students were more sensitive to the emotions of other people, more reflective about their own reactions, and better able to deal with ambiguous situations than men students. At the same time, some men complained about being assigned a female lab partner because "women are simply too emotional" and "doctors can't afford to be sensitive" (Hafferty, 1991). The tension physicians experience between empathy and detachment is very complex; ethicists increasingly recognize that traditional moral theory has underplayed "the importance of the 'emotional work' of life—of nurturing children, offering sympathetic support to colleagues, displaying felt concern for patients" (Little, 1996). Medical educators are paying more attention to how pressures on students to appear tough generate ethical dilemmas for students (Bickel, 1996); it is likely that women more than men suffer from these pressures and feel guilty about their emotional reactions to patients.

Studies of stress, in fact, do find that women medical students and residents experience more psychological distress than men do (Notman, Salt, & Nadelson, 1984). The reasons are many: Women in our culture tend, in general, to report more stress and less confidence in their abilities than men; women with family responsibilities experience role conflict and practical difficulties in managing all their responsibilities; and society undervalues women's careers compared with men's. Women students also experience more harassment from peers, supervisors, and patients (see Chapter 3). It is, therefore, not surprising that women medical students, more often than men, report worry about their academic futures and career decisions (Bergen, Guarino, & Jacobs, 1996). Reassuringly, however, women do not experience academic difficulty during medical school at a higher rate (4% of both sexes experience delay of graduation, leave of absence, or withdrawal or dismissal from medical school).

Do women students have any advantages over men? There is some evidence that women outperform men on obstetrics/gynecology rotations (Krueger, 1998). This might be because of access to clinical experience. In fact, some student affairs deans are concerned that because some women patients are refusing to allow men students to examine them, the education of men medical students on OB/GYN rotations is suffering.

Overall, differences between male and female medical students are better characterized as North Dakota/South Dakota rather than Mars/Venus. Basically, both men and women are people first!

Deciding on a Specialty

> I always wanted to be somebody, but I should have been more specific.
> —*Lily Tomlin*

In the United States, the largest proportion of women physicians currently practice in internal medicine (18%), followed by pediatrics (15%), family practice (11%), obstetrics/gynecology (8%), and psychiatry (7%). As shown in Appendix B, most of the new MDs who are completing residency training have likewise chosen these five specialties, in approximately the same proportions. Even though the number of women is increasing in all specialties, little change is occurring in the proportional distribution of women and men across specialties, with few women entering the surgical fields or any subspecialties. Many women are apparently still not finding mentors in or are discouraged from entering these areas, raising questions about whether women enjoy the same access as men to the full range of opportunities (even though they pay the same tuition).

Specialty choice involves many variables, so gender differences can be tricky to interpret. Men and women medical students give similar reasons for their specialty preference (i.e., self-fulfillment, positive clinical experiences, intellectual challenge). But as suggested by the AAMC survey results above, men give greater weight to financial factors in making career choices. Twice as high a percentage of women than men plan on locating in a socioeconomically deprived area (Bickel & Ruffin, 1994). Overall, women students are much more concerned about the problems of medically indigent populations and more likely to believe they are responsible for providing services to the indigent (Crandall, Volk, & Loemker, 1993).

Given the country's health needs, the increasing numbers of women physicians is obviously good news. But women should not automatically rule out any specialties choices. For instance, discussions with any of the 1,425 members of the Association of Women Surgeons will convince skeptics that surgery can be an absolutely fantastic career for a woman. In particular, women breast surgeons are in high demand. Women with breast cancer naturally prefer a woman surgeon to shepherd them through the emotionally and medically complicated process because a woman is more likely to sympathize with the dread of losing a breast.

Women do face extra hurdles in gaining respect in the still macho arena of surgery. For instance, women students might even be asked if they have the physical stamina to stand for the requisite number of hours (as if stamina were a Y chromosome-linked characteristic!). And some women students report feeling unwelcome and have trouble finding mentors and role models (Mutha, Takayama, & O'Neil, 1997). Dr. Frances Conley (1998), professor of neurosurgery at Stanford, just published an account of her experiences with sexism in the operating room, which are indeed cautionary. However, in part because of her very public stand against harassment, much progress is occurring in humanizing surgery and improving the educational climate in general (Bickel, Croft, & Marshall, 1996). So do not write off surgery just because of its negative mystique for women. Women patients deserve the option not only of a woman internist and a woman pediatrician, but also a woman surgeon. Plus, think of all the men who will be needing prostate surgery—the future of urology looks great!

Seriously, from the very beginning of medical school, it is wise to start thinking about specialty choice. The complexities of selecting a specialty, given the pace of technological change and the pressures of educational indebtedness, are escalating. But the key factor in specialty choice remains self-knowledge; this puts the ball in your court (see the section on Goal Setting in Chapter 4).

To help medical students with this whole process of selecting a specialty, AAMC teamed up with the American Medical Association (AMA) to develop MedCAREERS (see Appendix F). MedCAREERS is a career planning tool that begins with self-assessment and then explores specialties and decision making. This tool offers an exercise to explore the values that individuals find satisfying in their work; for instance, you rate the relative importance of such values as aesthetics, autonomy, security, spirituality, and compensation. You will also get help in assessing the skills you do especially well and those you especially enjoy doing (e.g., innovating, observing, motivating, visualizing, organizing). Financial planning is incorporated throughout each stage of MedCAREERS.

Once you've narrowed down your choice of specialty to one or two, you will start looking at individual residency programs. The AMA has created the Fellowship and Residency Electronic Interactive Database Access (FREIDA) online. This database allows you to define and prioritize various criteria to narrow your review of the 7,500 available residency programs.

Preparing for Medical School and Residency Interviews

Respondents to AAMC's Graduation Questionnaire report that residency directors ask women personal questions more frequently than men. Women interviewees are more likely to be asked about the stability of their interpersonal relations and their intention to have children. Women are also much more likely to be questioned about their commitment to medicine and about their spouse's support. Although some interviewers grill women applicants on their family plans with questions that make it clear there are no "right" answers, most interviewers are usually asking out of legitimate concern for program staffing requirements and want to know how the applicant prioritizes personal goals in relation to the demands of residency training.

Applicants naturally wish to please rather than alienate interviewers and should try to respond to all questions, even difficult personal ones. Therefore, *before their interviews* women applicants should prepare and practice answers to predictable personal questions, for example, about their plans to have a family (see also Chapter 2). And remember—after responding to questions about interests and goals outside medicine, especially relative to raising children— turn the conversation back to your commitment to medicine and to your academic and professional qualifications.

The following sets of questions will also help you prepare for your interviews.

- Three Questions You Will Probably Be Asked During a Medical School Interview

  1. What do you perceive as your weakness(es)? (This is a tricky question and one that requires finesse. Obviously "inability to make it to class" is unacceptable, while "compulsion to succeed" sounds like a weakness, but really is not.)
  2. What do you perceive as your strength(s)? (This will be your chance to sell yourself. Do not take up too much time answering this question, but at the same time, do not be afraid to assert your finer qualities.)
  3. Where do you see yourself in 5 (or 10) years? (Familiarity with your own goals and with the school's mission will help here.)

- Questions Commonly Asked During Interviews for a Residency

  1. How do you plan to use your training?
  2. How have you handled a patient with a particularly difficult personality? What did you do that seemed to help the situation?
  3. Discuss a stressful circumstance you had while in medical school. What made it stressful? How did you deal with it?
  4. Describe an instance when a professor criticized you for doing something inappropriately or incorrectly. How did you handle the criticism? What did you learn from that experience?
  5. What kind of working relationship have you had with nurses, technicians and other allied health personnel? What qualities do you think most contribute to teamwork?
  6. Can you foresee any circumstances that would preclude you from taking call throughout your training?
  7. How do you handle competing demands on your time?

8. What type of support system(s) do you have in place to assist you during your medical training?

9. How do you handle emergency situations? Give an example (Molidor & Barber, 1998).

- Three Questions You Should Consider Asking During an Interview
  (Note: Adjust these as appropriate for residency interviews.)

  1. Are there any special programs of which your school is particularly proud? (This will be the school's chance to sell itself to you. Be as knowledgeable as possible about the school's programs, and ask a follow-up question or two when appropriate.)
  2. What kind of academic, personal, financial, and career counseling is available to students? (A strong support system is not just fluff; it is a necessary component in medical education. Do not be afraid to ask about it.)
  3. How are students evaluated? (The grading system can radically affect the classroom environment. A pass/fail system often engenders more collaboration and less competition than the A through F method.)

Another possible resource to help you prepare for interviews is to be found at http://www.interviewfeedback.com where students fill out and submit questionnaires on their medical school interviews. For any medical school in which you are interested you may browse through remarks submitted by a wide variety of students over the past few years about their interview experiences.

A final tip: dress appropriately. Conservative is safest. Form-fitting, sexy sweaters will focus attention on qualifications that will work against rather than for you every time. Invest in a tailored, low-key suit. Wear flats or low heels. At the least, clothing should be perfectly clean, fit properly, and convey the messages you want conveyed about yourself (i.e., smart, confident, organized, professional).

Diagnose Yourself

(Note: This chapter contains answers, advice, or both on each of these questions, in the order they appear here.)

1. Does your undergraduate GPA look high enough for you to be a serious candidate for admission? What activities are you engaging in (or do you plan) that will assist medical schools in assessing your motivation for a medical career?

2. Where can you look up the admission criteria for each U.S. medical school?

3. Where can you find information on the numbers of women faculty and department chairs at each school?

4. What are some of the reasons that women medical students, in general, experience more psychological distress during medical training than men?

5. At this point what specialty interests you the most? Are there any resources available to help you decide what specialty might represent the best fit for you?

6. What kinds of questions should you practice answers to prior to your interviews for medical school and residency?

7. What clothes are most appropriate to wear for your interviews?

2 Medicine and Parenting

For Whom the Clock Ticks

> People who maintain a reasonable balance in their lives are more likely
> to maintain both their enthusiasm for their work and their self-respect
> better than those who risk burnout by sacrificing all else for rapid pro-
> fessional advancement.
>
> —*Kim Ephgrave, MD*
> *(1995, p. 3; former president of the*
> *Association of Women Surgeons)*

> Women are less likely than men to think that childbearing and child-
> rearing are someone else's job.
>
> —*Luella Klein, MD*
> *(first woman president of the*
> *American College of Obstetrics/Gynecology)*

This chapter begins with an overview of unresolved conflicts within our society stemming from the dominance of a male-defined work ethic. It then ad-
dresses the many practical questions that applicants and medical students (and
even residents and faculty) ask about balancing family responsibilities with the
educational and professional demands of medicine. Questions cover such areas as timing of children, responding to questions about childbearing plans,
breast-feeding, and exploring part-time options. The question and answer section explores "Can I have it all?" The last two sections offer some basics on
scoping out parental leave policies and finding child care.

Crosscurrents

Consider the many crosscurrents within Western culture regarding parenting, careers and traditional gender roles. Just 25 years ago, women were reading guides such as *How To Go To Work When Your Husband Is Against It, Your Children Aren't Old Enough, and There's Nothing You Can Do Anyhow* (Schwartz, Schifter, & Gillotti, 1972). Although a lot has changed in just one generation, most U.S. institutions are still organized around the myth that every household has a full-time mother at home (Coontz, 1992), and "working mothers" catch the blame for many societal ills (Hickey & Salmans, 1994). Double standards abound (e.g., when men do the dishes, it is called helping, and when women do them, it is called life).

Since both men and women display such a variety of orientations toward work and parenthood, why is the sexual division of parenting tasks that assigns emotional duties to women and economic duties to men so persistent? Why has the female culture shifted so much more rapidly than the male? The image of the "go-get-'em" woman has yet to be fully matched by the image of the "let's-take-care-of-the-kids-together" man (Rhode, 1997). Not as much positive change has occurred in the culture of home and workplace as one would have hoped from the sheer size of the social revolution that has brought women into the paid workplace in droves. In fact professional jobs seem to be structured to exclude the possibility of workers fulfilling daily commitments to family, home and community. One might ask why cannot society support *combining* paid and unpaid work as the adult norm? (Buchanan, 1996).

Any answers here are bound to be as complex as the questions. Penned by a medical school faculty member, *Dilemmas of a Double Life: Women Balancing Careers and Relationships* argues,

> Society has much to learn from our feminine values and ability to function within a relational context. Instead, women are often co-opted by the traditional male assumptions . . . [and] socialized to make life easier for others, we avoid the negotiations necessary to make life easier for ourselves. (Kaltreider, 1997, p. 30)

These large questions at the root of combining family and work are major societal issues. It is easy to be disappointed that obstetrician/gynecologists and pediatricians in particular have not surfaced as national and local leaders to improve family leave and day care. Unfortunately few physicians have worked to create a healthier way for the next generation. In fact, although this is changing, physicians who take time off for family risk being labeled as "uncommitted" (by patients and colleagues alike). Much patient care depends upon physicians' willingness to put their patients first, even when they are exhausted or overburdened. Indeed, the round-the-clock nature of patient care and the extended training period mean that medicine presents more challenges to raising a family than virtually any other career. For instance, as Lucy Candib (1995), medical director of a women's health center, writes,

> I found myself pitted against women with children. . . . I used my entrenched skill at denial not to hear what my women partners and residents were trying to tell me—that full-time was too much. . . . Caught by their feelings of responsibility toward each other and by their commitment to their patients, my colleagues persevered through years of insulting insinuations that because they had families they were unwilling to work hard enough. . . . But a stiff upper lip is the solution neither to overwork and fatigue nor to the complexity of multiple commitments. (p. 9)

Feeling like pioneers, too often women physicians have held themselves individually responsible for all the struggles involved, rather than working toward departmental and institutional solutions. Most women are fully occupied just trying to deal with all the practical aspects of balancing all the elements of their lives; one said she feels like an octopus with a candle burning at the end of each tentacle!

Part of the stress stems from the combination of two career clocks and two biological clocks. A high percentage (85%) of women physicians marry other professionals: 50% of those other professionals are physicians (Tesch, Osborne, Simpson, Murray, & Spiro, 1992). An even higher proportion (60%) of women *academic* physicians marry other physicians (Levinson, Tolle, & Lewis, 1989). A recent large study of married physicians with children found that 87% of the women and 62% of men experience at least moderate levels of role conflict between family and career (Warde, Allen, & Gelberg, 1996)— evidence that the men are sharing in more of the household responsibilities than their fathers probably did. Other evidence of change is that the younger men (49%) were nearly twice as likely as their older peers (28%) to have ever made a career change for marriage (e.g., a decrease in work hours). Nonetheless, many women physicians acknowledge that, while they have their partner's verbal support of their careers, they need more help with managing domestic responsibilities.

Although men are increasingly involved in their children's lives, it is women who have the primary responsibility for children. In a study of married pediatricians, women were twice as likely as men to state that family had affected career decisions. One man, compared with 274 women, interrupted his career for a family related reason (Brotherton & LeBailly, 1992). A major new study of physician faculty at 24 medical schools has found that women with children (compared with men and with women without children) obtained less institutional support (e.g., secretarial assistance), and had fewer publications, and lower career satisfaction. No significant differences on these and other variables were found between men and women without children (Carr et al., 1998). Most women physicians expect tradeoffs, however, few choose to have lower salaries or less administrative support than their male colleagues with similar professional responsibilities.

A "dual-career" family actually has four ticking clocks: two biological clocks and two career clocks. Plus, there are all the rest of life's little responsibilities (e.g., when the water heater breaks, the kids are sick, the dog needs shots, the mortgage must be refinanced, not to mention food shopping, dinner, dry cleaners, etc.). Among other problems, these four ticking clocks spell S-T-R-E-S-S on the relationship (Sotile & Sotile, 1998). Thus, it comes as a breath of fresh air for one prominent physician-couple (formerly co-editors of the *Annals of Internal Medicine*) to declare: "the old way of demanding single-minded dedication to medicine needs to be recast because it depended on a full-time backup for the rest of life's activities" (Fletcher & Fletcher, 1993, p. 628). Some leaders within the profession understand that "women physicians, insisting on being fair to their families, are trying to lead the profession toward [a more] balanced life" (Bulger, 1998, p. 110).

Although superwoman died of exhaustion at some point in the 1970s, many women currently in medical school seem to have missed this news. One Harvard student writes,

> Perfection. Medicine expected it. We demanded it. We may fail in our first attempt at Mount Success. But we'll spend the rest of our lives trying . . . [and] we applied the same exacting standards to our personal lives as we did to our academic pursuits. (Rothman, 1999)

Many women learn the hard way that the superwoman strategy backfires. A University of California San Francisco professor of clinical psychiatry (Kaltreider, 1997, p. 137) comments about many of the young women professionals seeking psychotherapy: "Like the ancient deities, they feel that they can carry the full potential of both sexes. Inevitably this perception collides with an inhospitable workplace, a biological limitation, or a limiting relationship, and an agonizing reassessment is often the result." The message here is: Strive to set reasonable goals and reassess them frequently.

There are obviously no easy solutions to facilitating balance for physicians. It is wrong to conclude that medicine and parenthood are incompatible. Although physicians do face extra challenges in integrating their personal and professional lives, most have a huge advantage: a comfortable income that can buy a lot of help. Moreover, most physicians (especially in primary care) discover a synergy between parenting and evolving as a clinician. Certainly the experience of having and raising a child enormously expands a physician's appreciation of the miracle of birth and of the physiology and psychology of pregnancy, gestation, and children's developmental stages—not to mention family dynamics and preventive health issues. Moreover, consider the numerous likely areas of transfer of learning between the personal and professional lives. Clinicians who are parents will have, for example, heightened awareness of people's need for praise and acceptance of failure. They'll also hone their organizational and time management abilities and the skills of managing multiple roles, collaborating, and managing conflict.

The rest of this chapter can actually be considered "preventive medicine" (no, not birth control). The following sections answer as honestly as possible the questions most commonly raised about combining family and career to give you a clear picture of the terrain. This is a first step in charting your own path through it. Once you start looking, you will find good examples of physicians who have both happy families and successful careers who can give you pointers along the way. Remember most women physicians can expect about 30 years of professional life after their children are in school, though for many that life stage will entail attending to the needs of parents as well, but that's another story!

Common Questions Medical Students Ask About Combining Medicine and Parenting (and Some Answers!)

When is the best time to start a family? Young women (and increasing numbers of men) entering medicine frequently ask this question up front. About 80% of medical students intend to or already have children (Osborn, Ernster, & Martin, 1992). An assessment of the hopes and concerns of one medical school's first-year students found that family issues topped the list of concerns for both women and men; almost one third of all concerns students expressed fell under the category of the effect medicine will have on marriage, children and other personal relationships (Fields & Toffler, 1993).

The answer about timing is, of course, "it all depends"—on God, your partner, your age and health, your support system, your finances, your career goals. Because of the demands and stress of new clinical responsibilities, the hardest time to be pregnant may be the first year of residency. A close second may be the third year of medical school, depending on the amount of flexibility your school can allow (and on whether your student loans will come due if you take significant time off). However, numerous women have successfully accomplished both pregnancy, child care, and training responsibilities during even these intense years of clinical training.

A study of pediatricians found that men had an average of 2.6 children and women, 1.7; residency was the most common time of the birth of the first child. This study found that the women who became board certified were more likely to postpone childbearing until after training (Brotherton & LeBailly, 1992). Another survey of pediatricians revealed a median age of 29 at which they had their first child; residency years were reported as the best time for pregnancy. In retrospect, 58% indicated they would have chosen the residency training period again to have their first child but 36% would have chosen an earlier time (Sells & Sells, 1989). A study of women internal medicine faculty revealed that, of the women who were currently married or had been married, 79% had children. The mean age at the birth of the first child was 30.6 years and at the birth of the second, 32.9 years. Seventy-nine percent of these women faculty with children reported breast-feeding their infants for an average of 6.5 months; 81% returned to work while doing so. Forty-six percent of the respondents with children had their first child after completion of training. Almost three-quarters reported being satisfied with the timing they had chosen (Levinson et al., 1989). Thus, studies of physicians show that most do realize their plans to have and raise a family.

What about the health of physician-mothers and their children? The largest study of residents found that 29% of women residents experienced at least one pregnancy during residency; 8% voluntarily terminated the pregnancy, but 78% of pregnancies resulted in live births (Klebanoff, Shiono, & Rhoads, 1991). This study found that in spite of the women residents' long hours (an 80-hour work week is not unusual), they were *not* at greater risk of spontaneous abortion, when compared with wives of male residents. However, these women did experience slightly higher rates of preeclampsia and premature labor (Klebanoff, Shiono, & Rhoads, 1990). Another study similarly found that despite sleep deprivation and increased stress, female residents were as likely to give birth to a full-term newborn as the spouses of male residents (Osborn, Harris, Reading, & Prather, 1990).

A study of male and female residents whose families experienced a pregnancy during residency found that neither sex missed much work because of pregnancy (fewer than 7 days per trimester). Not surprisingly, residents' wives took much longer maternity leaves (15.5 weeks) than female residents (5.8 weeks) (Harris et al., 1990).

And then there are the new stresses. For instance, some experience loneliness in dealing with the challenges of parenthood. Many have worries about finding and keeping child care (Kiely Law, 1997). As residents attempt to balance a demanding call schedule with child-rearing, some feel guilty about any special treatment related to a pregnancy and responsible for any resentment from colleagues who work extra hours due to their abbreviated schedules (Wiebe, 1997). Some overcompensate by working "equally long shifts to prove that they are 'good' residents" (Chow, 1997). Juggling the roles of parent, spouse and physician, especially under tight financial constraints, is certainly a challenge (Turk, 1997). But the result is usually positive and a very rich life.

What else does a physician-in-training need to think about in regard to starting a family? Stating the obvious, child rearing is a huge responsibility. Here are some questions that might help in thinking through the decision to start a family:

- What are the maternity and paternity leave provisions?
- What is the availability of assistance with child care? Is having a child caretaker who speaks the same language as you important to you? What is the minimum age of children that day care facilities in your area accept? What are the longest hours of operation of your first choice child care facility? Is there a waiting list? What resources are available when your child is sick?
- Can you rely on members of your family to help?
- How much additional debt will child care expenses entail?
- The early years of parenting are especially precious, and some mothers and fathers end up regretting not being more present for the "first" everything. How willing are you to give up some of these opportunities?

What about "medical" marriages? Unfortunately, women physicians are at higher risk for divorce than their male colleagues. A large study of Johns Hopkins University graduates found that women physicians were more likely to divorce than their male colleagues, particularly women in psychiatry and surgery (Rollman, Mead, Wang, & Klag, 1997). However, there's good news from the largest database ever assembled—the Women Physicians' Health Study ($N =$ 4,501)—which revealed that women physicians are more likely to be married and less likely to be divorced than other U.S. women (Frank, Rothenberg, Brown, & Maibach, 1997). This study corroborates previous findings that physicians' marriages are less likely to end in divorce than those in other occupations (Doherty & Bruge, 1989).

As previously noted , a high percentage of women physicians marry other physicians. And most physicians who are married to other physicians find that sharing their professions as well as their lives is highly enriching on many levels.

The other side of the coin is that "medical" marriages, especially if either partner is still in training, are at risk of expiring from general fatigue and lack of attention. Relationships require work and nurturance. When both, or even one partner is suffering from chronic fatigue, the couple may stop communicating effectively. Severe problems can develop in short order.

It is helpful to explore some of the dynamics involved. Medical students learn to delay gratification, thinking life will be wonderful when they finish training. Once out of training and married, many cannot turn that behavior off and continue to focus mainly on work, delaying the "gratification" of a home life. Moreover, physicians also tend to be Type A personalities who have a hard time slowing down and listening to others. One consultant comments:

> While Type A's are among the happiest and [most] successful people, the stressed Type A's accumulate frustrating experiences and become Type Aggravated. What with? Type B, B, B, B! As in: Move your Big slow Behind out of my way so I can get about my Business and lower my Blood pressure! (Linney, 1999, p. 82)

Some words to the wise:

- Because life (and any partnership) ends up being far more stressful and complex than anyone can anticipate, renegotiate cooperatively, lovingly, and periodically your relationship contract.

- Ignore minor irritations if you expect peace and harmony.
- If you can't get away together for long, take minivacations. Set limits on the extent to which you are available to patients and colleagues.
- View vulnerable feelings as powerful resources rather than weaknesses to be overcome; view setbacks as learning experiences and stressful times as necessary steps toward desired goals.
- When things are not going well, apologize and empathize.
- Seek out experiences that will help you continue to grow in healthy directions.
- Consider the equivalent of "well baby check-ups" and go for counseling every few years whether you think you need it or not (Linney, 1999).

Here is a final word of advice from a book on medical marriages: "When the ethic in your marriage is that you are two good and imperfect people who are trying your best to manage your life, your relationship becomes a place to grow" (Sotile & Sotile, 1998, p. 162).

How should medical students respond to program directors' inquiries about their personal lives and childbearing plans? The law prohibits discrimination in hiring decisions on the basis of sex (including pregnancy), and questions pertaining to family plans may be evidence of impermissible discriminatory intent. Candidates are not required to answer them; and if a program does not select a resident, the fact that the questions were asked can be offered in support of a claim against the program. If a student feels that an interviewer is overly aggressive in pursuing questions, she may contact the federal Equal Employment Opportunity Commission or the state agency that handles discrimination claims.

Despite the illegality of such questions, applicants naturally wish to avoid alienating interviewers at residency programs on their wish-lists. Therefore, as is also covered in the last section of chapter 1, before your interviews, prepare for predictable personal questions. Practice articulating your values and goals in a strategic and convincing fashion; it helps to ask a friend to role-play a hard-nosed program director interviewing you.

Women who hope to have a child during residency or who are uncertain of their plans need to think very carefully about how their responses may be received. Most program directors have experience with residents who claimed not to be considering pregnancy but who did become pregnant during training (or arrived pregnant!); these program directors are now suspicious of other residents "misleading" them. Although a few program directors carry their probes too far, most pose their questions about family plans out of legitimate concern for clinical staffing needs.

Prospective residents can use these inquiries to find out how supportive the program director is, how the leave policies work, and how absences are handled. You can gain crucial insights about whether this program is a good fit for you. You can also demonstrate to the program director that you understand that a resident's absence has implications for the program.

In any conversation about your family plans, however, you should turn the conversation back to your commitment to medicine, to your academic qualifications and to your career interests. Immediately after their interviews, students who are uncomfortable about anything that occurred should write down their memories of what transpired so that they have a record for possible later discussion with a student affairs dean or hospital administrator.

What about breast-feeding? Many states now have legislation barring discriminatory practices regarding breast-feeding—giving mothers a right to breast-feed and to legal recourse if denied (Baldwin & Friedman, 1998). For example, in Connecticut it is now illegal to restrict or limit a mother breast-feeding her child in a public place. In Florida, public sector employees must be provided written policies supporting Breast-Feeding practices in the workplace (i.e., flexibility in work schedule for milk expression, accessible locations allowing privacy, close access to a clean, safe water source and sink for washing hands and breast-pumping equipment, and access to hygienic storage).

In 1997, the American Academy of Pediatrics (AAP) issued a policy statement on Breast-Feeding and the Use of Human Milk. Two of their twelve recommendations are particularly pertinent for medical schools and teaching hospitals in accommodating lactating mothers: (a) Develop and promote policies and procedures to facilitate breast-feeding (e.g., electric breast pumps and private lactation areas, both on ambulatory and inpatient services), and (b) provide (and allow without penalty) adequate time for employee-mothers to breast-pump (AAP, 1997).

La Leche League International is a nonprofit organization with headquarters in Schaumburg, Illinois (see Appendix F). They provide education, information, support, and encouragement to women who want to breast-feed. La Leche League also provides continuing education on breast-feeding and lactation management for physicians. There are over 3,000 local La Leche League chapters across the United States which provide telephone counseling 24 hours a day, pertinent literature, parenting support groups, and mother networking.

Support for breast-feeding mothers is becoming more common. Depending on the setting, most hospital units or clinics already have a refrigerator in which you could store breast milk; check with the unit or clinic supervisor to be sure this is okay.

What part-time options are available? First of all, "part-time" has an altogether different meaning for physicians than for the layperson. Because patients need help at all hours, it is not unusual for physicians in practice to work 60 hours a week, and residents may be in the hospital more than 80 hours. Therefore part-time may mean 35 or 40 hours, which is full-time in most work settings. Even so, individuals seeking a less than full-time residency must proceed with great care, because most program directors are seeking residents with a full-time commitment to the program, their own training, and their patients. However laudable and human it is to have small children during that interval, many program directors and other staff physicians will interpret a reduced schedule (even for family responsibilities) as a lack of commitment to medicine.

Nonetheless, if you have small children or other immediate responsibilities, and need more flexibility than a full-time schedule permits, by all means seek a residency that will allow you a part-time year or more—especially if you are a strong candidate. First check with your specialty boards to see if there is a policy limiting part-time training. For instance, the American Board of Family Practice allows part-time residencies, as long as the resident maintains the usual schedule continuity. That is, although the resident might be on rotation at the hospital only half-time, she still would have a full load of office patients (Wilke, 1999). The next step is finding a residency program where a reduced schedule is feasible. Unfortunately, no centralized resource on this subject exists. In general, reduced schedules are most likely to be arranged in large residencies and in primary care fields, and most difficult in small programs and in surgery.

Another possibility is to seek a "shared-schedule" residency, where two residents share one residency slot and salary. The specialty board should be able to tell you which programs have recently offered this as an option. If this sounds good, during your residency interviews, if not before, explore this as a possibility. The trick here is finding someone with whom to share the position; this would need to be a person with whom you can develop the highest level of trust and cooperation.

Once in practice, it is generally easier to find or create a part-time or shared job. In a shared job, each partner works part-time, usually fewer than 25 hours per week in the office, and shares rounds, call responsibilities, and so forth with another physician—often a spouse! Some might work four half days; others prefer two or two and one half very full days. Downsides are reduced income, half days turning into full days because of paperwork and time spent updating the partner, and less clinical experience than full-time physicians (many part-timers try to make up for fewer cases with more time spent reading medical journals).

Individuals negotiating a part-time job position should be especially careful with their employer to get everything spelled out in writing (e.g., malpractice coverage, continuing medical education leave-time, vacation benefits, on-call terms).

"Can I Have It All?" Choosing medicine as a career means also choosing extra challenges in leading a balanced life. As pointed out earlier, superwoman died of exhaustion. Everybody has limitations on their energies, their health, their relationships—not to mention a workplace that doesn't exactly match their specific plans and goals! So how do you set reasonable expectations?

For one thing, realize that sacrifice is a necessity. Although the hoary-headed in medicine wax eloquent about the pains and joys of sacrificing themselves for their patients, entering students tend to be more focused on the "self-actualization" aspects of a medical career and to worry about carving out time for their family or for personal pursuits. Every physician finds her own spot on this continuum between self-denial and self-actualization (they are not really opposites). But many medical educators (and admission committee interviewers) worry that too many students have unrealistic expectations about "having it all"—as if it were possible to be the excellent physician they see in their mind's eye as well as the devoted parent, loving spouse, and organized manager of all of the rest of life's responsibilities, without sacrificing something, somehow, somewhere. (Hint: the first thing to go is usually any exercise program or creative endeavor.)

Self-care and self-esteem are very closely linked. When you cut back on time for exercise, friends, and hobbies for many years in a row, you burn out. You might experience a growing sense of meaninglessness that can turn into clinical depression. Most people can bounce back, but not always and not in all arenas. Juggling is a good metaphor: Some balls are fragile and crack when dropped (e.g., your relationship with your child or partner). Other balls bounce back (e.g., a failed test can be retaken, most health problems are short-term). For each person, the degree of fragility and bounce will vary with each of the balls in the air, but no one can keep them all in the air for long!

Difficult choices and tradeoffs are inevitable no matter what path you are on—and a full life is full of tradeoffs. The way is seldom straight and the trajectory is seldom a steady line up. Because of their multiple roles and longer life spans, women professionals have wavier trajectories than men (Bateson, 1990). Despite all the possibilities now open to women with high aspirations, there are few examples who model balance or who demonstrate pacing themselves evenly across a long life span. The main message here is, without selling yourself short or shortchanging your patients, do not try to do too much at once. With regard to your professional goals, think long-term. Sometimes what appear to be hindrances and detours can become the basis for life's greatest lessons about what is important.

It may help to think in terms of "5-year plans" of relative emphasis. For instance, if you already have a child, consider taking an extra year for medical school. If you are just completing your residency and want an academic career, you might plan on devoting the next 5 years to establishing your research program and clinical reputation, and then for the subsequent 5 years, having a child and working 50% or 75% rather than 100%.

Parental Leave Policies

Slowly over the past few decades, America's institutions of higher education and hospitals have been developing fair policies to guide administrators when a student or employee has a child (Bickel, 1989). In previous eras, women having children were more likely to drop out of school or work, or to expect no leave. Although women trying to balance challenging work with family responsibilities still have to forge their own solutions, a pregnant woman who expects to remain active and needs temporary accommodation is no longer a surprise!

Students are paying to receive an education, and the question of "leave policies" is altogether different from an employment context. Usually a student's need for flexibility in the curriculum is addressed individually by the appropriate medical school administrator. In most schools the number of women students having children is small enough that their needs for flexibility are usually accommodated without special policies. Students with loans who take leave for more than 1 year at a time need to be aware of possible complications. For instance, a student who uses up her 9 months grace period might need to begin repaying some loans prior to returning to student status.

For residents, policies regarding time off and benefits vary a lot. And taking all the time off allowed by a policy will entail sacrifices. The most important actions for you to take are the following: (a) find out what the policy is as soon as or before you are pregnant, (b) try to predict how your absence will affect your schedule and others, and (c) give administrators as much advance notice as possible. Problems occur when women err on either end of the spectrum (i.e., they assume they have no rights to accommodation and leave, or they presume that everyone should accommodate their pregnancy- and child-rearing-related needs in a generous spirit). Some women undermine colleagues' otherwise-available support with an air of entitlement. Do not expect extra understanding from a female as opposed to a male administrator because each woman makes different choices regarding child bearing and child rearing.

If you want to start a family during residency, look for large training programs that usually have more flexibility to modify schedules (Iserson, 1996). For example, a residency program at the University Hospital of Cleveland deliberately assigns "jeopardy" duty to a few residents who can be called to fill in for residents who have a family or personal emergency (Wiebe, 1997).

Once you are in the program, schedule less demanding electives during the months surrounding your baby's birth—perhaps those for which you would have no overnight responsibilities (Wiebe, 1997). Also, seek out any existing campus resources or guidebooks for employees on child bearing and child care.

Policies for Students

In 1992, Case Western Reserve University School of Medicine established an ad hoc committee to address needs that some students have for flexibility in the curriculum. The committee recommended several ways in which to allow for maximum flexibility without jeopardizing educational goals: Make information about the challenges of balancing personal and educational responsibilities available to all students; encourage faculty to recognize and avoid biases in evaluating students seeking flexibility; and suggest that each department prepare a written decelerated curriculum to allow for uniformity and clarity in implementation. The committee also suggested a revision of student leave policies to include flexible options such as extended clerkships (allowing for 50% more time) with an educationally equivalent workload, short leaves between clerkships, or an opportunity to take certain core clerkships in the fourth year.

Student leave policies at medical schools tend to allow two categories: short periods of one month to one semester, or longer periods of 1 to 2 years. Student absences almost always require the dean's approval; however, at some institutions course directors may approve absences of 30 days or less. Leave may be granted for personal, medical, educational, or family reasons. Personal leave might be granted to a student reconsidering medicine as a career choice, but most institutions have strict guidelines about when and how students might choose this option and require students to provide a detailed justification for such. In most instances, medical leave is granted for mental or physical illness or conditions which interfere with medical school. Students returning from medical leave are usually required to present evidence of health clearance from the student health service to their dean's office. Educational leave may be granted to students pursuing research or other degree programs. Family leave is normally granted in two circumstances: for maternity or paternity responsibilities or for the death or serious illness of an immediate family member.

Policies for Residents

Most teaching hospitals now have written policies for maternity leave, parental leave, or both (Philibert & Bickel, 1995). In the most recent study (conducted in 1994) 41% of teaching hospitals reported dedicated *paid* maternity leave, with a mean of 42 days allowed (although many women do not take this amount of time). Twenty-five percent allowed paternity leave, and 15% adoption leave.

In 1993, 86% of eligible family practice residents completed a survey on their experience of giving birth during residency. The average length of maternity leave was 8 weeks; 75% had leaves of 10 weeks or less. For many, the maternity leave was derived from multiple sources, including vacation, sick time, or a mother-child elective. Nearly all (88%) the women breast-fed and the mean duration of breast-feeding was 19 weeks. The problems most frequently encountered after their return to work were sleep deprivation, difficulty arranging for child care, guilt about child care, and breast-feeding (Gjerdingen, Chaloner, & Vanderscoff, 1995).

The American College of Physicians has recommended that a parental leave policy for residents include the following minimum elements:

- Guidelines for length of leave allowed before and after delivery
- Procedures for requesting leave

- Procedures for alteration of leave due to an unanticipated event or complicated delivery
- Whether salary and benefits are provided during leave (for example sick time, vacation time, short-term disability)
- Whether time absent needs to be made up in order to fulfill requirements of the certification process
- If residents are required to make up additional months, whether they will receive benefits and salary during this time
- If leave is extended, whether the institution or the individual must pay health insurance premiums
- Whether accrual of vacation and sick time continues during parental leave
- Whether flexible planning (for example, returning to work part-time) is available
- Whether the policy applies to adoption and paternity leave (Levinson, 1989)

The Family Medical Leave Act (FMLA) of 1993 applies to most residents. The FMLA requires employers with 50 or more workers to grant up to 12 weeks of unpaid leave each year to new fathers and mothers (including adoptive parents) who have worked for at least one year.

Remember that a leave policy is just the beginning. A lot of planning between residents and directors is still required to minimize disruptions. Adding staff to replace absent residents adds costs. Residents who take all the leave available to them may be subject to criticism from unsympathetic colleagues and may also face concerns about the adequacy of their training. Finally, specialty boards' requirements vary regarding time allowed during residency for maternity or disability leave. Therefore, residents should check to make sure their board's requirements are not more restrictive than their residency program's.

Child Care

Child care resources in academic medical centers remain limited. Only 46% of major teaching hospitals offer on-site child care for children of housestaff physicians. And the majority of these facilities are only open 8-12 hours per day (many fewer hours than a resident's typical day). Only one quarter of these have services for sick children. Of those institutions offering on-site child care, 60% reported that demand for child care exceeds their center's capacity and the average waiting time is seven months.

A few medical centers have notable programs. Children's Hospital Medical Center in Cincinnati has an on-site child care facility in the Department of Pediatrics called Children's for Children; it is open every day of the year. Yale University's Phyllis Bodel Childcare Center was originally conceived and organized by women faculty and postdoctoral fellows at the School of Medicine; it is named in honor of Dr. Bodel, who was the first director of the Office of Women in Medicine at Yale, the oldest such office in the country. Children of parents affiliated with the Yale School of Medicine and Yale School of Nursing receive priority. A scholarship fund assists the neediest parents.

In 1998 Harvard University's Office of Work and Family produced a 70-page *Family Resource Handbook* (President and Fellows of Harvard College, 1998) filled with information on pregnancy and postpartum resources, choosing child care, finding a babysitter, as well as resources related to caring for older children and the elderly. The guide even includes an appendix on activities to do with children around Boston and important legal and tax information. Although the guide's focus is the Boston area, it does include some national resources and topics important for any physician-in-training to consider when starting, raising and caring for a family.

The American Association for Women Radiologists (AAWR; see Appendix F) recently produced a small booklet, *Child Care: A Combined Experience from the AAWR* (Rosenfield, 1998) in which members share their experiences with child care. Contributors address topics such as nannies, child care at meetings, single mother dilemmas, and firing a caretaker.

Although still far from optimal, resources and support for physician-parents are increasingly available. More and more leaders within medicine recognize that "opportunities for mutual growth of individuals and families can be fully realized only when the profession truly recognizes the importance of families" (Beiser & Roberts, 1994, p. 1673).

Diagnose Yourself

1. If you have a partner or significant other, how do you anticipate she or he will adjust to the increased hours you will be devoting to your education and responsibilities? Who will take the lead in managing domestic responsibilities?

2. Although physicians face extra challenges in making time for family, what are some of the upsides for physicians with regard to bringing children into the world?

3. Along the continuum from the first year of medical school to the first year of practice, when is probably the hardest time to be pregnant?

4. How will you respond to program directors' inquiries about your child-bearing intentions?

5. What health concerns might you anticipate if you become pregnant during your residency (when an 80-hour work week is not unusual)?

6. If you become pregnant, how will you handle the implications for your fellow residents, given that your absence will translate into longer hours for them? What help can you expect from your hospital's parental leave policy?

**Sexism:
The Eye of the Beholder**

The more a woman is perceived as a woman the less likely it is that she will be perceived as professionally competent.
—*Virginia Valian (1998, p. 136)*

"That's a pretty good dissection, for a girl." "You're much too cute to become a urologist." "Be glad to give you a free physical exam." To some women such comments are little more than a joke, and they reply in kind. Other women get angry, others frightened, and others disgusted. Still other women might take as little note as a duck does to a little shower. This range of possible responses illustrates the "eye of the beholder" characteristic of most kinds of harassment and sexism. Such remarks also reveal an enduring antagonism toward women that is not uncommon in many cultures. How to respond to remarks such as these remains a challenge for most (Bickel, 1997).

Sexism is defined as the belief that one sex is superior to the other (Tronto, 1995). Although both sexes may joke about women's claiming superiority, female chauvinism has *not* affected men's economic or social status. Male chauvinism negatively impacts women in multiple ways (and no one jokes about it). When feminists coined the term "sexism" in the 1960s, many expected that, with women gaining long-denied rights and entering male-dominated professions, sexism would die a natural death. But the legacy of historical oppression is tenacious, and women continue to experience sexism as a delegitimizing force, rather like a "ton of feathers" (Caplan, 1993).

A great deal of progress has been made since the days (just a generation ago) when women medical students faced open hostility and charges that they were "taking a man's place." Today, overt hostility and demands for sexual favors in exchange for continuing employment are illegal. The sexism that remains is actually subtler than before laws were on the books—and in many ways therefore harder to address.

Sexual harassment is the most serious and addressable manifestation of sexism. We begin with data from recent studies in medical school, residency and practice, followed by examples of how individuals and institutions can put a stop to harassment. Next we discuss the problems with students dating supervisors (consensual sexual relationships). In the final section we probe how gender stereotypes continue to interfere with women's professional development and offer suggestions on overcoming these negative effects.

Harassment: The Evidence

> Before sexual harassment was given a name, women called it life.
> —*Gloria Steinem*

The courts, universities, and other organizations have promulgated a broad array of definitions of sexual harassment. However defined, sexual harassment is primarily a manifestation of *power* rather than sexual attraction. In environments and organizations which heavily emphasize hierarchy, as in the military, harassment of those low on the totem pole is not uncommon. Unfortunately, medicine falls into this category.

The most intensive and meaningful studies of sexual harassment in medical education have been conducted by individual schools. For instance, at Stanford University, a 1994 survey of medical students revealed that women students (46%) experienced significantly more sexually harassing behaviors than men students (15%). Asked whether they had observed sexual harassment, 70% of both women and men students reported observing at least one of the following behaviors at least once: negative sexist remarks or jokes, stereotypes portrayed in presentations or lectures, demeaning public displays, offensive gestures, or passive support of such behaviors (Bergen et al., 1996). Students who experienced or observed any of these behaviors were more likely than the other students to rate the educational environment negatively, thus for most students even overhearing an attending physician tell a sexist joke detracted from the educational experience.

Sexual harassment in medical education does appear to be decreasing—as would certainly be expected given all the publicity and work focused on this problem in the last decade. For instance, the proportion of fourth-year medical students at the University of Toronto reporting sexual harassment decreased from 36% in 1991 to 22% in 1994 (Moscarello, Katalin, & Rossi, 1996). Similarly, 22% of women and 3% of men graduating from medical school in 1996 reported being subjected to offensive sexist remarks or names directed at them personally; these proportions were higher in 1992. Clinical faculty and residents continue to be the biggest source of the problem, followed by fellow students (Kassebaum & Cutler, 1998). A 1996 study of 1,001 students at eight medical schools corroborates the above results, with 20% of women and 2% of men reporting verbal sexual harassment (Mangus, Hawkins, & Miller, 1998). But 41% of both sexes reported nonsexual verbal harassment. Clearly medical education remains a long way from the "zero tolerance" of harassment that is proposed by many institutional policies.

Looking beyond medical school, problems remain at the housestaff level as well. A study of internal medicine residents at the University of California-San Francisco found that three fourths of the women and one fourth of the men had been sexually harassed at least once during training. Of those harassed, 79% of the women and 45% of the men believed that harassment created a hostile environment or interfered with their work, but only two women and no men reported it to an authority (Komaromy, Bindman, Haber, & Sande, 1993). The lack of reporting is certainly one of the reasons for the continued prevalence of harassment; the reasons for this reluctance are discussed in the next section.

Another study asked residents in 13 residency programs at the University of Toronto and McMaster University about four kinds of abuse and discrimination. No gender differences were found with regard to psychological and physical abuse. Psychological abuse from attending physicians was reported by 68% of both men and women, from patients by 79%, and from nurses or other health workers by 77%. Forty percent of both women and men reported an instance of physical assault from patients. Seventy percent of women respondents reported gender discrimination from attending physicians, 88% from patients, and 71% from nurses; for men, rates were much lower (23%, 38%, and 35%, respectively). Women also encountered sexual harassment more often than men from attending physicians (35% vs. 4%), from peers (30% vs. 6%), and from patients (56% vs. 18%) (vanIneveld, Cook, Kane, & King, 1996).

Studies of physicians in practice likewise continue to be very concerning. Focusing first on harassment from patients, a study of women family physicians in Ontario found that more than 75% reported some sexual harassment from patients (Phillips & Schneider, 1993). Despite their power as physicians, some women physicians find that their male patients treat them more as women than as physicians (i.e., the vulnerability inherent in their sex sometimes overrides their power as doctors). A survey of 1,400 physicians in Canada found that women more often than men physicians reported gender discrimination not only from patients (women 67%; men 13%), but also from peer physicians (56%; 6%), from senior physicians (48%; 5%), and from nurses (44%; 9%) (Cook, Griffith, Cohen, Guyatt, & O'Brien, 1995). Finally, a new study of over 4,500 U.S. women physicians who graduated from medical school between 1950 and 1989 found that 48% had at some point experienced gender-based harassment and 37% experienced sexual harassment (Frank, Brogan, & Schiffman, 1998). Women in historically male-dominated specialties (e.g., surgery) or employed by a medical school reported a higher prevalence of sexual harassment. This study also found that women who are divorced or separated and those who are less satisfied with their careers were more likely to experience harassment. Of greatest concern is the finding that the younger the physician, the more likely she was to report harassment during medical school; this finding may reflect a heightened general sensitivity to sexual harassment or may indicate that even as late as 1989 there were no improvements to the training milieu.

Putting a Stop to Harassment

Many individuals who are harassed experience anxiety, fatigue, eating or sleeping disorders as a result; education suffers and in some cases so does the person's commitment to medicine. Patient care is ultimately affected. These costs and losses and the multifaceted nature of the problem mean that a variety of initiatives are called for (i.e., educational programs, preventive measures, and policy development).

Virtually all higher education institutions and hospitals now have a policy pertaining to the reporting and handling of sexual harassment (Sandler & Shoop, 1997). Most policies distinguish between *quid pro quo* harassment (decisions or expectations based on an employee's or student's willingness to grant or deny sexual favors) and *hostile environment* harassment (unwanted conduct of a sexual nature has the purpose or effect of unreasonably interfering with an individual's work or academic performance or creating an intimidating or hostile academic or work environment). Most policies tend to be fairly complex because of legal ramifications and because due process is paramount in protecting the rights of both accused and accuser. Trainees need to know where to find the policy if the need arises; in most cases it will be printed in the student handbook or readily available from the dean's office. The Accreditation Council for Graduate Medical Education (ACGME) now requires residency programs to include in the resident's employment contract an outline of specific policies and procedures whereby complaints of sexual harassment are to be addressed.

Medical students are understandably fearful of "rocking the boat" or negatively affecting one of their clerkship evaluations. They need multiple mechanisms for coming forward with complaints, with confidentiality ensured at all stages for both accuser and accused. Because perceptions of harassment are so variable, institutions must take a great deal of care in defining and addressing them (Nora, Daugherty, Hersh, Schmidt, & Goodman, 1993).

A policy on the books will not go far in eliminating poor behaviors if members of the educational community are ignorant about what constitutes harassment or are too fearful to report incidences. A proactive program of prevention education and complaint resolution must be in place (Hippensteele & Pearson, 1999). Some medical schools distribute educational materials annually. For instance, Yale University School of Medicine's pamphlet, titled *Tell Someone,* (1998) describes what constitutes sexual harassment and how to go about reporting it. The pamphlet's primary messages are that you should not blame yourself and that you should not remain silent.

Another promising institutional avenue is the appointment of an ombudsperson, a neutral individual hired to resolve concerns or conflicts and to remain objective and treat all parties equally. For example, Yale University School of Medicine's ombudsperson serves several roles: (a) *neutral complaint-handler* to insure that people in the medical school community are treated fairly and equitably (any troublesome matter in the community may be discussed), (b) *conflict manager* to solve problems through mediation and informal third-party intervention, and (c) *mediator* to provide a locus for the discussion of troublesome matters in the community (Waxman, M., personal communication, December 4, 1998). Yale's Ombuds Office is independent of other administrative structures, maintains confidentiality, and keeps no formal written records.

Likewise, Harvard's Ombuds Office offers students, residents, faculty, and staff a "safe place to get help" with interpersonal concerns or conflict, including sexual harassment, racism, professional misconduct, stress or anxiety, working conditions, or favoritism.

In terms of changing behaviors, evaluation mechanisms are as important as resources and policies. But the evaluation of faculty as role models of profes-

sionalism and respectful behaviors remains far from routine. Many faculty unfortunately feel justified in perpetuating a standard of behavior to which they
became inured as students, and some abuse the immense power imbalance in
the supervisor-trainee relationship. Students should have the opportunity to
evaluate their faculty, residents and attendings on a "professionalism scale"
(i.e., how they treat their colleagues and trainees) (see also Chapter 5). For
instance, each clerkship evaluation would ask students whether the faculty
treated them and others with respect and whether faculty demonstrated any
sexist or racial bias. This would provide students a relatively easy mechanism
for reporting, say, a preceptor who calls them "honey" or a resident who makes
sexual jokes.

A focus on prevention of harassment is key. In every appropriate way, deans
and faculty should stress civility and professionalism in the learning environment. Unprofessional behaviors in educational institutions are public problems which ultimately require institutional solutions.

As for individual responses, here are some options for handling a problem
yourself:

1. *Use humor:* You could say in a somewhat joking manner, "Is this a test to
   see how I react to sexual harassment?"

2. *Give one back:* If someone calls you "honey," you might say "that's Dr.
   Honey to you!" This kind of humor connotes strength and makes it clear
   that the comment did not accomplish the belittlement intended.

3. *Name or describe the behavior and indicate your disapproval:* "That comment is offensive, it is unprofessional, probably is sexual harassment and
   has to stop."

4. *Pretend not to understand:* Especially useful with sexist jokes, keep a
   deadpan expression and say, "I don't get the point" and then ask the person
   to repeat the joke, continuing to claim a lack of understanding.

5. *Write a letter to the perpetrator:* First, document in a factual manner what
   happened, without any evaluative words. Second, describe your feelings
   about the incident, such as, "I find it very offensive." Finally suggest what
   should happen next, for example, "I expect to be treated in a professional
   manner." The letter is typically sent certified (return receipt requested).
   Keep a copy of the letter but do not send it to anyone else. This method is
   usually successful but may not work with a hostile or sadistic person.
   Once in a while the harasser wants to apologize or explain, but just reply,
   "I don't want to discuss it, I just want the behavior to stop" and walk away.
   This approach gives the harasser an objective view of her/his behavior
   (Sandler & Shoop, 1997).

What can individual women students do when the difficulty is with a patient? Because physicians-in-training are still learning the boundaries of the doctor-patient relationship, how do you tell appropriate from inappropriate behavior, and then how do you set firm limits? These skills take time to acquire. It is important for all physicians to learn to differentiate among types of patient comments and to be prepared to handle inappropriate or abusive ones. For instance, if a patient calls you a "dish" you should not hesitate to reiterate your professional role and your expectation that the patient address you with respect (Justice & Mulrow, 1995). If the patient repeats the offense and for more severe types of disrespect, you may have to seek assistance from a superior.

In general if you feel uncomfortable with a patient's behavior, pay attention—the patient may be crossing a boundary. Do not shy away from talking about the issue directly with the patient, and do not let the problem build. At the same time, learn to *depersonalize* incidents—you did not cause the problem; but by not dealing with the problem expeditiously you may contribute to its continuation (Phillips & Schneider, 1993). You pay a great price for not trying to fix the problem, however.

"Consensual" Sexual Relationships

An example of a "consensual" relationship in medicine is an attending physician dating a medical student. Such relationships are controversial. Many believe that such relationships are nobody's business (some even result in happy marriages). It is not always clear who initiated the relationship. Another wrinkle (however unfair) is that some men "blame" their women trainees for being attractive; unfortunately the self-esteem of many young women depends on their being sexually desirable and they may welcome the attention of a man with status (Lane, 1998).

There are, however, good reasons for policies against consensual sexual relationships—primarily to prevent vulnerable students from being taken advantage of by individuals with a lot of power over them and with responsibilities for their evaluation. Such relationships often skirt the boundaries of abuse of power and are therefore a professional conflict of interest (Lane, 1998). Whether or not there is a policy at your institution forbidding such relationships, it is wise for women to steer clear of dates with individuals above them in the hierarchy, no matter how limited the "eligible partner" pool may sometimes seem.

Overcoming Gender Stereotypes

As muddy as sexual harassment issues can be, problems with gender stereotypes tend to be even murkier because of their subtlety. Stereotypes are percep-
tual shortcuts. We all acquire them from our families, early education, and societal messages. Children's books contain unwitting sexist messages; a study
of recent children's literature found that male characters still come up with solutions eight times more often than females (Rhode, 1997). Going back to the
books your mom read as a child, how many women characters can you find
who are not princesses, witches, or happy housewives in aprons? A large body
of research reveals that, when asked to rate scientific articles, works of art, and
curriculum vitae, both men and women evaluators tend to give higher ratings to
work ascribed to men than to women (Sandler, Silverberg, & Hall, 1996).

Actually research on "right to die" cases involving incompetent adults reveals an extremely serious manifestation of gender stereotypes. One study
found that judges respected men's personal autonomy to a much greater extent
than women's (Miles & August, 1990). The study concluded that women were
disadvantaged because their moral agency was taken less seriously. Because
we do not see people as "gender-neutral" but rather as male or female, women
lose out a lot of the time without even being aware of it.

Gender role expectations used to be much starker than they are now (e.g.,
women actually used to believe they should be seen but not heard). But they remain powerful influences. For instance, compared with men, women are still
expected to be less ambitious and assertive and more patient, compliant, and
ornamental. Individuals who act "against type" (e.g., men who are emotional
and women who are aggressive), are suspect. Even husbands of women leaders
do not escape ridicule; when the press asked former British Prime Minister
Margaret Thatcher's spouse who wears the pants in his family, he responded, "I
do, and I also wash and iron them" (Jamieson, 1995). Consider as well how so-
called universal plots do not work when the sex of the protagonist is changed
(e.g., "a young man puts his business career first and loses his masculinity, end-
ing up a lonely eunuch)" (Barreca, 1991).

Women still face a number of double binds that men do not. Women who
are too feminine will be judged incompetent, and women who are too competent, unfeminine. Also, as men age, they gain wisdom and power; as women
age, they wrinkle (Jamieson, 1995). Another kind of double bind relates to a
new trend with regard to showing emotion: Bob Dole got positive points from
the press for tearing up when he announced his decision not to return to the
Senate, but when Pat Schroeder wept during a similar announcement, her tears

were interpreted as a sign of weakness, as in "what can you expect from a woman?"

Because of the ways it can interfere with their progress, women need to understand the inherent (though seldom stated) conflict between "femininity" and "competence." Compared with boys, most girls are still taught not to be too assertive around men, and throughout their lives are allowed a much narrower band of assertive behavior. Further implications of these phenomena are discussed in greater depth in Chapter 4. A final point here is that gender stereotypes also influence students' evaluation of faculty. If women professors are not nurturing, students judge them much more harshly than they do men professors who are not nurturing; that is, students' expectations (perhaps for an ideal mother) interfere with their fair evaluation of the merits of these women faculty (Sandler et al., 1996). Women medical students are sometimes angered and often disappointed to find that the few women surgeons on the faculty may be as macho and demanding as the men faculty; the students are unthinkingly but understandably holding the women faculty to a higher standard than the men.

Women who are ethnic minorities experience additional challenges. When something unfairly negative happens, they ask themselves "Would this have happened if I were a man? Would this have happened if I were white?" (Secundy, 1996, p. 121). African American women medical students participating in a focus group responded to questions about their ethnic and gender identity, academic performance, and stress. Several racially based stressors emerged, including isolation, alienation, and negative assumptions about intellectual abilities, with many of these women reporting that they often felt compelled to prove themselves worthy and intelligent. Gender issues became prominent in clinical rotations when several were mistaken for nursing or other allied health personnel (Shervington, Bland, & Myers, 1996). An African American woman writes of her experience at Harvard Medical School: "There were never any overt racial incidents . . . [but several times] it was clear I was obviously invisible . . . [and] one patient made no bones about not wanting a black student-doctor caring for him" (Blackstock, 1996, p. 78). This physician also cites a number of examples of the difficulty both African American and Caucasian people have in seeing African Americans in roles of authority. Hispanics encounter similar dilemmas.

Gender and ethnic stereotypes also interfere with physicians diagnosing and treating patients (Schulman & Berlin, 1999). Physicians, because they are more powerful than patients, may never even learn they are biased because power and stereotypes reinforce each other; dominant persons (especially those who are attentionally overloaded) tend to ignore information discrepant to their stereotypes (Fiske, 1993).

The "eye of the beholder" phenomena also adds to the difficulty of addressing stereotypes and sexism. The following oxymorons illustrate the slippery nature of many incidents (Benokraitis, 1997):

- *Collegial exclusion:* The head of the lab asks only the guys to lunch.
- *Radiant devaluation:* A faculty member compliments a medical student on her hair instead of on her highly competent report.
- *Friendly harassment:* Women medical students announcing an American Medical Women's Association meeting are ridiculed with joking catcalls from male students.

What can you do to overcome the negative affects of gender stereotypes? A no-brainer is to steer clear of men who blame women for having to watch their jokes and their hands. Most importantly, realize that double binds and microinequities reflect *systemic* bias and are not a reflection on you. If you do not appreciate the systemic and cultural nature of these stereotypes, you may blame yourself and question your competency. Such competency-doubting reinforces women's tendency to attribute failures to internal causes (e.g., lack of ability); men tend to attribute their failures to external causes (e.g., a difficult situation) (Geis & Butler, 1990). At the same time, take care to dress and act professionally; if your clothes or voice are sexually suggestive, then you are asking for harassment.

Few forums exist for men and women to jointly consider these problems. Easily threatened men label women who raise these issues "dykes," "whiners," or "weak sisters." Equally unfortunate is when women accuse men of bias when they ask legitimate questions. Respectful listening—from both sexes— is necessary for common understanding.

Individually, you must hone your conflict management skills (see Chapter 4) and become braver and more direct in responding to sexist comments (see suggestions in the previous section). It is also essential to identify secure men who, with some encouragement, will stand up to their peers' sexist comments. You can draw on your network for support and for advice regarding which battles to fight. One excellent network is the American Medical Women's Association (AMWA) which has student chapters in most areas. One AMWA resource is a Gender Equity Information Line, offering telephone advice to women physicians, residents, and students experiencing gender discrimination or sexual harassment (see Appendix F).

Framing sexism as one of many problems of student mistreatment, AAMC's Organization of Student Representatives (see Appendix F) created a series of vignettes illustrating common forms of mistreatment. This exhibit, titled "Drawing the Line on Student Abuse," invited participants to indicate whether or not abuse was occurring in the example (e.g., "Sara was rotating through OB/GYN. In the OR, the attending asked her what she wanted to do. Sara respected this attending a lot and was proud to say that she wanted to become an OB/GYN. He looked at her and said, 'You know you look more like a pediatrician.' ") (Cohen, 1999, p. 45).

Many schools are addressing problems with unprofessionalism head-on. For instance, the University of Virginia's School of Medicine's Medical Student Advocacy Committee distributes information annually to all students and faculty on how to report sexism, racism, sexual and racial harassment, racial discrimination, verbal abuse, or other types of unprofessional or offensive behavior; the Committee confidentially investigates all reports. In addition to such advocacy efforts, some schools are making room in the curriculum for serious discussions of sexism and gender stereotypes. Cases illustrating these subjects can be included in required or elective bioethics, professionalism, and social issues courses (see Appendix C). The goal of all these efforts is an educational environment in which women's presence and contributions are as valued as men's.

Diagnose Yourself

1. What forms of sexism in our culture most affect you?

2. What do you think you would reply if your anatomy partner, with a serious face, said *"That's a pretty good dissection, for a girl"?* Would you respond differently if the comment came from a peer with whom you did not have to work so closely?

3. How would you respond to a patient who calls you "honey?" Would the age and sex of the patient matter to you?

4. Do you know how to find the sexual harassment policy at your medical school?

5. What are some of the problems and risks involved with dating a faculty member?

4 Beyond Survival: Maximizing Your Professional Development Options

> Learning is the ability to enhance one's capacity to accomplish something one really cares about.
>
> *—Peter Senge (1999, p. 190)*

It is never too early to begin blue-skying your future as a physician, especially if you really want to make a difference in the world. This chapter assumes that you have high goals, that you have a lot to contribute and that you want to progress as far as you can. We begin with food for thought about why so many fewer women than men have progressed into senior ranks in medicine. In order for this reality to change, more young women must make a lot of wise career moves and develop their capacities to the fullest. The second section offers suggestions on the seldom-discussed process of setting professional development goals. The last three sections concentrate on exceedingly important skill areas with which many women need help: self-presentation, conflict management, and job-related interviewing and negotiating.

Cumulative Disadvantages

> Ironically, women who acquire power are more likely to be criticized for it than are the men who have always had it.
>
> *—Carolyn Heilbrun*

Although the number of women is increasing at every level in medicine, women at the top are scarce (see Appendix B). The "average" U.S. medical school has only 19 women full professors (that's about one per department) and only about 5% of academic clinical departments are chaired by a woman.

New studies shed some light on why women are not progressing to the top in greater numbers. After 11 years on a medical school faculty, 23% of a national sample of men but only 5% of women had achieved full professor rank (Tesch, Wood, Helwig, & Nattinger, 1995). These women had the same preparation for an academic career as their male peers, but they began their faculty appointment with fewer academic resources (e.g., protected time for research, lab space, research assistants). Another study found that men and women's research and academic productivity were equivalent, but women faculty received less compensation and were less likely (33%) than men (47%) to attain the rank of full or associate professor (Carr, Friedman, Moskowitz, & Kazis, 1993). Another cohort study found that women faculty were less academically productive and spent more time in teaching and patient care than men. Although women represented 35% of respondents, women accounted for less than 20% of the "highly productive" respondents; compared with highly productive men, these women reported a poorer quality of mentorship, less adequate institutional support of their research, and less overall career satisfaction (Kaplan et al., 1996). The final study of note to be mentioned here found that women physician faculty with children (compared with men and with women without children) obtained less institutional support and had fewer publications and lower career satisfaction (Carr et al., 1998).

Thus, the picture is complicated. Men tend to outpace women in the venue counting most toward promotion in academic medicine (i.e., research and publication). Men also are more likely to obtain the mentoring and to negotiate the resources necessary for academic career success. Even when they are as qualified and productive as men, women are less likely to reap the rewards. So we see at work a complex combination of inhibiting factors, including sexism and cultural stereotypes (see Chapter 3), lack of mentoring (see Chapter 5), and family responsibilities taking time and energy (see Chapter 2). The following deals with those factors less easily classifiable into one of these chapters.

"Cumulative disadvantages" offers a useful construct for considering why women are not progressing in pace with men. Beginning at the beginning, we do not perceive people as "people" but as males or females, and comparisons almost always disadvantage females (Valian, 1998) (see Chapter 3). It is also inescapable that in terms of role models for careers, men are advantaged by growing up surrounded by examples of men who have changed history, made laws, and led countries. By contrast, most middle-aged women in our culture learned to read from a primer in which Jane helped her mother clean while Dick climbed trees and had adventures.

Moreover, men continue to have "company" as they enjoy career success. As a woman progresses, she becomes a greater and greater rarity and thus lives in a "glass house" where she is always highly visible and there is no room for error. This kind of stress begins well before a woman or minority reaches the top; any nontraditional member of a previously homogeneous group tends to be subjected to more intense scrutiny and to quicker judgments.

Another subtle cumulative disadvantage faced by successful women is that they make insecure men uncomfortable. A survey of women executives in Fortune 1000 companies asked the women the reasons for their success. The top two answers were "consistently exceeded performance expectations" and "adjusted personal style so it would not threaten male executives" (Decade of the Executive Woman, 1993, p. 3). In other words, successful women learn to alter their behaviors to avoid making male colleagues uncomfortable. Men tend to be most comfortable with women who smile and defer to them. To keep from being described as having "sharp elbows," women must often tone down their styles.

Men rarely even need to think about this extra skill set. But women must take great care. To achieve one's goals, one must be "adequately aggressive," that is, "take initiative, defend oneself when attacked, recognize one's goals and be able to plan one's life according to them" (Cantor & Bernay, 1991, pp. 59-60). Women who are not adequately aggressive will be ignored or discounted. But in most cultures women have a narrower band of assertive behavior than men enjoy. Men seldom have to choose between competence and masculinity, whereas women still face many potential conflicts between competence and femininity. The same behavior that is considered laudably "goal-oriented" or "competitive" on the part of a man is often labeled "harsh" or "confrontational" in a woman. No wonder there are so many jokes (often bitter) about women bosses. In order to gain respect, an authority must be serious; but any woman who tries to speak authoritatively runs the risk of being seen as humorless, taking herself too seriously, and labeled "uppity" or worse (Tannen, 1995).

Our culture's lack of experience with women as idea-generators is also why women frequently do not get credit for their ideas. Many laugh at a cartoon showing a woman sitting at a conference table surrounded by men, with the leader saying "that's an excellent suggestion, Ms. Jones—perhaps one of the men here would like to make it." Virtually all women professionals report that in meetings ideas they suggest are often credited to a nearby man or to a man who later repeats their idea. Women are also more frequently interrupted than men in meetings. Even though men belittle these phenomena, women get tired of and angry at being treated as if they are "transparent" or "invisible." Do not ignore being ignored, it will sap your energy and commitment. Also, a big component of professional advancement is the ability to parlay small gains into bigger ones. It is important to get credit when credit is due even if it seems like a "molehill." A light touch and diplomacy are necessary when "correcting" anyone, and battles must be chosen carefully. But keep in mind that mountains are molehills, piled on top of each other (Valian, 1998).

The root of these phenomena are complex. Carol Gilligan (1990) studied how the exuberant voices of nine year old girls become the carefully regulated self-presentation of adolescent girls. As they enter puberty, many girls' self-assurance goes underground; in conformity to social pressures, self-confidence plummets. In contrast adolescent boys remain likely to say that they are clever and able. Gilligan concludes that the "construction of a feminine sense of identity goes counter to the leadership skills and intellectual competence necessary for success in the workplace" (p. 25). This difference in orientation is illustrated by a telling modifier in the Girl Scout oath. Whereas the Boy Scout oath states: "On my honor I will do my duty," Girl Scouts say: "On my honor I will *try* to do my duty."

Finally, although demands on time are intense for all medical students and physicians, many women receive additional demands beyond those relating to family and personal responsibilities. Women are more likely than men to be asked to do things not in their educational or career interests (such as acting as secretary at a meeting or running an errand for someone). Women tend to accept the "caretaker" roles because of their socialization and because they are "conflict averse." Men seem to be better at setting boundaries and regarding the pursuit of their own individual goals as justified. Women experience both practical and psychological difficulties to closing the door and tuning others out.

These disadvantages are presented as a map of the terrain—not to discourage anyone from the hike. The better you understand the lay of the land and how far your predecessors have come despite grave difficulties, the more likely you are to succeed.

Let's close here with a mention of an obvious "cumulative *advantage*" for career success that many men have. They begin and stay centered in a "careerist" orientation; that is, they remain focused on what will advance their career. It is not surprising, for instance, that men scientists see science as a vehicle for financial stability and professional status to a greater extent than do women scientists (Sonnert & Holton, 1995). Women's orientations tend to be broader and more community and family focused, and less focused on external rewards.

Although they are changing, societal expectations of men as breadwinners and women as caretakers still do influence career orientations. These societal stereotypes do not work to the advantage of either sex. Although many men are ambitious, some suffer from the expectation that they devote themselves to work, even if they prefer a life centered around family. In fact men have fewer "normative alternatives" than women, who may devote themselves to caretaking, breadwinning, or any combination.

Goal Setting

If you don't know where you're going, you are likely to wind up someplace else.

—Casey Stengel

The first goal of medical students is to graduate and obtain a good residency. This section will be of greatest use to young physicians in residency who are planning their next steps. Because the health care environment is increasingly competitive, the "random" method of career planning is unlikely to provide satisfactory results. It is never too early to set personal and professional goals for yourself. Goals are both your destination and the guideposts for your career (Wolf, 1998). And it's worthwhile to write them down. The mind is a very messy, forgetful place; the process of writing brings its own clarity. Retain your drafts and notes; they'll become a very interesting and telling record of your own maturation.

Managed care necessitates more managed careers (see Chapter 6). Although older physicians bewail increasing restrictions on their professional autonomy, medicine still abounds with positive choices and rich opportunities. Apply a prevention and fitness model to your goal setting: values-driven and holistic, allowing balance and integration with your personal life, and requiring periodic evaluation (Pearson, 1998). Or think in terms of designing your own car—instead of just choosing options, like the color, imagine what your "ideal car" would look like—and go for it! (Whitfill, 1998).

One of the pitfalls for women is a *job* focus instead of a *career* focus. There is a lot to be said for focusing on the intrinsic rewards of the task at hand, but it is also important to have a long-term perspective with an eye on future benefits. A "job focus" radically increases the likelihood that after 20 years of hard work, you will find yourself discontented and disappointed without understanding what went wrong.

Here are some suggestions to get you started in your goal setting and forecasting:

- You may be putting too much of the burden on your well-developed left brain and not giving your creative, nonverbal right brain a chance for input. Try for a "middle brain" intelligence, a fluidity that allows a questioning of your usual assumptions, and take a fresh look at the world.

- Try "scenario building" with a creative, forward-looking friend. Imagine a series of "what ifs" with regard to the environment and your own development.

- Try "PMI" (plus, minus, interesting) to help you drop a static mind-set. Take any problem you are considering and create a column of answers to the questions: "What about this is Positive?" "Negative?" "Interesting?" (James, 1997).

- Remain curious, live "in" your questions rather than "against" them—in your personal life as well as your professional life (Flower, 1999).

Physicians do face more difficulties than other professionals in integrating their careers with a healthy personal life (see Chapter 2). With the 24/7 work ethic in medicine, it is a real challenge to incorporate personal goals into your career planning. You need support; it is almost impossible to accomplish this combination on your own. Find others with the same general values and find a way to work together. No longer in short supply in most locales, physicians have more freedom to limit their hours if they choose. A big part of the problem is mind-set:

The model of a successful life that is held up for young people is one of early decision and commitment to an educational preparation that launches a single rising trajectory. . . . These assumptions, however, have not been valid for many of history's most creative people and are increasingly inappropriate today. Improvisations can become significant achievements and insights arise from the experience of multiplicity and ambiguity. (Bateson, 1990, p. 5)

Begin by asking yourself what gives you the most energy, what makes you want to get out of bed in the morning? To what ideals and personal goals are you most committed? What do you want out of life? What do you want out of your work? How do your life and work goals fit together? Do they mainly reinforce or challenge each other?

The "perfect job" mirrors the person who holds it; find, invent or create such a job by linking who you are with what you do. This process depends on your developing clarity about your talents, passions, values and the type of working environment that supports what you care about most (Leider, 1995). Except for the very charmed, this process occurs mainly by trial and error; but remember: Chance favors the prepared mind!

Begin with where you want to be in 5 and in 10 years (it is helpful to think in terms of "five-year plans" of relative emphasis). If you draw complete blanks, don't be discouraged (but keep reading this section). Once you have a good idea of your goals, plan the steps which will lead to their achievement. Start by asking yourself: What skills will I need? Should I undertake any extra responsibilities now to prepare myself? What about my marketability? What am I good at that is in demand now and will become more so?

Setting time aside (perhaps monthly for short-term goals and yearly, on your birthday or New Year, for long-term) to review your goals reminds you of where you're headed and why, and provides an opportunity for you to assess your priorities and needs. Consider using this COPE criteria when reviewing your commitments:

- *Critical*—must be completed for career success
- *Obligatory*—not critical to personal success but mandatory for your work team
- *Preferable*—enjoyable but not required for professional success
- *Extraneous*—unnecessary for personal or professional development (Wolf, 1998).

Of course, you'd want to spend more time focusing on the Critical and Obligatory commitments, and from time to time, reevaluate the necessity of those you consider Preferable or Extraneous.

Feedback is the breakfast of champions. Talk over your plans with someone you trust, if possible someone more advanced (this is one of the main functions a mentor can serve; see Chapter 5). Ask them to consider whether you are being realistic in your aspirations and to honestly evaluate your skills and background relative to your plan. Are you underestimating or overestimating your potential? Have you taken into account your weaknesses and problem areas? Although asking for a critique can be difficult (never ask a question you don't actually want the answer to), encourage your evaluators to be as specific as possible with regard to their perceptions of your strengths and weaknesses. Then take what you hear with a grain of salt, depending on the source.

Here is some additional advice:

- Seek challenging assignments with the greatest variety and number of lessons and that motivate you to learn. Look for assignments that are very relevant to current problems in health care.

- Keep your eye on the horizon for trends in what the population is seeking in health care and get involved (e.g., creating a woman-physician-run practice that offers extended hours and all types of alternative health care).

- Most physicians need to acquire many skills not covered in medical or graduate education (e.g., to challenge assumptions about yourself and your career, to communicate with a diverse and empowered team without being "in charge," to understand cash flow and financial statements) (Haid, 1998).

- Learn to recognize when your stress level has maxed out. If you just keep pushing yourself, you will likely end up depressed or ill, and your bad temper and poor judgment may irrevocably damage important relationships. Everyone reacts to stress differently, so finding your most effective way to handle stress takes exploration (e.g., if you react with headaches, try yoga, deep breathing, meditation, or exercise).

Life is unpredictable; the most careful plans can collapse. Adaptability is essential. But rather than encouraging the acquisition of such traits as adaptability and flexibility, college and medical school shield young people from work-a-day realities, actually delaying the development of survival skills (e.g., planning ahead, managing a budget, paying bills). These delays can result in damaging default on commitments. The clearer your thinking about where you want to go and the more firmly planted in realities, the more effectively you will be able to evaluate your options at each decision point, and the wiser your choices will be.

Finally remember that progress may not be steady or speedy. All rising is by a winding stair, and women's paths tend to undulate more than men's because of their multiple roles and responsibilities.

Self-Presentation

Nothing great was ever achieved without enthusiasm.
—*Ralph Waldo Emerson*

Effective presentations are beautiful compositions, virtually seamless, disguising the amount of preparation entailed. Excellent writing and speaking skills require much work behind the scenes, including assessing your audience's needs, organizing your materials, and creating visual aids. The only aspect of this process that is addressed here are suggestions for developing *self-presentation* skills. Fortunately, many resources are available on the other components (Mindell, 1995; St. James, 1996; Tannen, 1995).

As discussed above, some women must tone down their styles to be maximally effective. A more common need, however, is for women to strengthen their self-presentation skills because they are too soft-spoken, emotional or indirect to win serious consideration.

Whether speaking or writing (we're talking about professional communications here, not letters to mom):

- Do not start sentences with *I* unless you are talking about yourself. Instead of "I think we need more time," simply say, "We need more time."
- *Feel* is a four-letter word; avoid it unless the subject under discussion is your feelings (which are—like it or not—usually irrelevant in interviews and presentations).
- Trim hedges (i.e., do not hide behind phrases such as "I guess"). Do not say something if you do not mean it; if you mean it, you are not "guessing."
- Do not apologize if you have nothing to apologize for. For example, if approached about a new responsibility, rather than "I'm sorry but I'm not sure," say "I am interested but will need some time to consider it."

When making any kind of presentation, whether to one person or to a small or large group, remember that your body and gestures reveal much about your level of confidence. You are seen before you are heard, so consider ways in which you can strengthen your body language to give a positive first impression. Acquire a "posture of power": stand up straight, hold your head high, maintain eye contact, and smile unless a poker face is more appropriate. Avoid slouching, unnecessary movements, gripping a podium, clenching your fists, playing with jewelry or notes, and touching your hair (Mindell, 1995).

Your vocal characteristics—tone and speed—are important too. A squeaky, breathy or high-pitched voice weakens your message; a voice coach or speech pathologist can help address these and other problems. Take care not to speak too quickly, especially when you are nervous; do not be afraid of pauses and silence. Before you begin speaking, relax your belly and breathe as deeply as you can (rather than quick, shallow breaths). This technique will also relax you; in fact relaxing your belly is an excellent way to keep tension from accumulating in your body during difficult conversations and meetings.

There's no substitute for practice. Before an important interview or presentation, consider taping yourself (voice, video, or both) and getting feedback from a close friend.

Finally, always be on the look out for effective women and men to emulate—and there are lots in medicine. Study those you admire and incorporate elements that work for you. Soon you will have developed your very own effective self-presentation style.

Conflict Management

> It is provided in the essence of things, that from any fruition of success, no matter what, shall come forth something to make a greater struggle necessary.
> —*Walt Whitman*

Another essential skill is the ability to manage conflict. All the inherent sources of conflict in medicine are becoming more intense, and everyday life presents numerous opportunities for conflicts to arise. Many people misperceive conflict as a disruption of order or a sign that a relationship has gone sour; this is particularly true of individuals from families where conflicts were suppressed or where angry blaming frequently occurred (Siders & Aschenbrener, 1999). Actually, conflict is a natural consequence of growth and diversity. Its periodic occurrence can be healthy in relationships as an opportunity to clarify goals and values (Weeks, 1992). Unfortunately, many women tend to avoid conflict or to immediately accommodate the other person; such avoidance and accommodation not only interfere with their effectiveness but can also limit the growth of relationships.

Many women have some unlearning to do. Consider the games children play. Girls' play is characterized by sharing so that everybody can win; no one wins at dolls or acts as boss (for long). Girls tend to avoid conflict that can damage relationships and actually downplay ways in which one child is better than another. With parents frequently admonishing their girls to "be nice," girls learn to keep the power "dead even" so there are no winners or losers; their games continue indefinitely with rules made up as the play proceeds (Heim, 1993).

By contrast, in most of their team sports and rough play, boys emphasize their own ascendancy, learn to relate to each other through conflict, and challenge others in order to improve their standing in a group. In their games, boys deceive other players by pretending to have the ball; in most girls' games deception is disgraceful. In sum, girls seek to "get along"; boys to "get ahead."

It is not that one of these modes is better or worse than the other. But experience with sports and rough play (or maybe it's just the testosterone) does seem to make men more comfortable with competition than women are. Team sports does provide an excellent training ground for success in most American workplaces (Heim, 1993). Team sports, such as football and baseball, teach which rules are nonnegotiable and how to put aside individual goals for the purpose of winning. In sports, players posture aggressiveness even when they do not feel it; this offers practice with bluffing and putting the goal ahead of fears. Players obey the coach without question, learning how hierarchy and rules operate. Most players lose 50% of the time, so they also get practice at dusting off and regrouping after failure.

Understanding how games are played and how rules operate is essential to effective conflict management. So, if you do not have much team sports experience, or if your family of origin taught you that anger is wrong and conflict is bad, it will probably take you longer than many of your male colleagues to comfortably manage conflict. In addition to avoiding and accommodating, which obviously do have their place sometimes, you will need to develop the three other main conflict-management styles: competing, collaborating, and compromising (Thomas, 1992).

As you practice competing, collaborating, and compromising, you will get better and better at sensing which conflicts call for which modes. As you learn, resist the impulse to replay criticism to yourself. Guilt is a useless emotion. Learn what you can and move on. Also resist the urge to cry when your feelings are hurt; even though tears are very natural, they can be interpreted as a sign of weakness. A handy tip: jutting your chin forward usually stops the flow of tears. Cry later. It does have a healing effect.

Finally, remember that a mistake is an event which you have yet to turn to your full advantage. Experience is the best teacher. Think of your practice as snorkeling: from the surface of the ocean you can guess little about the rich life underneath. Once you take advantage of opportunities to "snorkel" within any club or organization's culture, you gain crucial insights into how it operates and into how to improve your self-presentation, conflict management and negotiating skills. All of this will help you "lean into" and draw on your considerable personal power, so that you can be as competitive or collaborative as you want to be!

Job Seeking, Interviewing, and Salary Negotiations

> Obstacles are what you see if you take your eyes off the goal.
> —*Anonymous*

Here are a series of generic suggestions for thinking through the job search process; most are applicable to both faculty and practice positions (see Chapter 1 on interviewing for medical school or a residency). The goal is to stimulate you to prepare a template of your needs and to be as thorough as possible in researching whether the position meets them.

- Update and review your curriculum vitae to be sure that it effectively and honestly reflects your accomplishments.
- Do not drag your feet in exploring and applying for positions that interest you. Investigate physician employment Websites on the Internet.
- Identify the journals advertising the type of position you seek and routinely review them (ask your librarian for advice). For example, *Academic Physician and Scientist* (a collaborative effort of medical publisher Lippincott Williams & Wilkins and AAMC) provides bimonthly recruitment news and classifieds in academic medicine.
- Consider who you know who will hear of the kind of job you want and talk to them. In some cases you will want your mentor to nominate you.
- Ask people senior to you who know you well if they will be comfortable acting as a reference. Ask them if they can give you a favorable recommendation.
- If you submit your curriculum vitae to a number of places but do not get invited to visit, try to elicit feedback as to the credentials of your competition and why you lost out. Try to ascertain if your goals are unrealistic and if you need to revise your plans.

Strategies for interviewing include the following:

- When invited for an interview, prepare as thoroughly as possible. Learn as much as you can about the institution and the position. Consider what questions you will be asked and rehearse your answers. What do you have to offer and why are you an excellent candidate?
- Dress professionally. A dark suit is no longer an iron standard, but conservative colors are safest. Conservative accessorizing is also best because you do not want anything to distract the interviewer from your professional qualifications (Heim, 1993).
- Do not be intimidated by the interview situation; do not be too modest about your accomplishments but never exaggerate. Carefully observe the culture.
- On a second visit, seek as much clarity as possible about responsibilities, expectations, constraints. Find out as much as you can about your boss and the fiscal situation. Look for clues about the culture, including whether the careers of women and minority members are thriving. Try to get all of your questions answered.

Salary determination is a complex institutionally-determined process. Within a residency program, salary levels are set within the hospital, however, the Accreditation Council for Graduate Medical Education (ACGME) requires institutions to provide reasonable compensation (financial and benefits). For most other jobs and positions, it is important to understand how the salaries are funded, how much negotiation room you have, and whether men or women are paid equally. Do not shy away from research about the organization's finances. And do not be a victim of math anxiety! If you understand the basic terms, reading a balance sheet is no harder than following a gourmet recipe and is certainly easier than interpreting an X-ray!

The best and most recent gender analysis of earnings found that young male physicians earned 41% more per year than their female counterparts; in medical school practice settings, the average income for men was $129,000 per year compared with $101,000 for women (Baker, 1996). However, after adjustments for specialty, practice setting, hours worked, productivity (i.e., patients seen per hour), educational variables, experience, characteristics of the community, specialty-board status and other characteristics, few earnings differences between men and women were evident. Men with 10 or more years of experience and those in internal medicine subspecialties and in emergency medicine still earned more per hour than women. In family practice, women earned more per hour than men.

Smaller studies show that equity appears to be slower in coming to the surgical specialties than to primary care. A recent study of cardiothoracic surgeons, after controlling for age and years of postsurgery experience, found no gender differences in training backgrounds, numbers of publications, hours-per-week worked, or proportional divisions of time among professional activities (Dresler, Padgett, MacKinnon, & Patterson, 1996). But half of the women reported a salary markedly less than the men; these differences could not be explained by academic rank, hours worked, or publication rates. One likely explanation is that the women did not negotiate their salaries. A study of cardiologists found that with regard to their first jobs, women were much more likely than men not to have negotiated any important job features such as salary, benefits, travel, space, support staff, or administrative duties (Limacher et al., 1998).

Believe it or not, some women are still told that they do not need a higher salary because their husbands are so well-paid. Women are indeed held to different negotiating standards than men are. Men are expected to be "hard" negotiators when a lot is at stake; one who does not actively assert himself may be considered a "wimp." Whereas, as discussed above, a woman risks being considered "too big for her britches," if she negotiates aggressively. No wonder many women do not press hard enough to get their due! But if a woman accepts a lower offer than she has to, she not only sells herself short but her employer concludes (a) that she's not an effective negotiator and (b) that she is actually only "worth" the pay she accepted.

There are many other job features to negotiate in addition to salary, including flexibility in your schedule and less-than-full-time options, which are of paramount importance to many women at points in their careers. The desire for more time with their families is certainly one reason why women's salaries are lower than men's; flexibility and time off are more important than salary to them. Although this difference in values is completely defensible, women must nevertheless avoid being taken advantage of simply because they shy away from discussions about money or do not know how the negotiating game is played.

A couple of final words here. Beyond salaries, negotiating a contract, especially for your first job, can be complicated—especially if you're dealing with a non-physician-run managed care organization. Before you sign on, do your research (Fox, 1998), talk to your lawyer friends or, better yet, to colleagues who have aced the process themselves.

Developing excellent negotiating skills is a lifelong process that is never too early to begin. Here are some of the most accessible and best books:

Negotiating for Dummies (Donaldson & Donaldson, 1996)

Negotiating at an Uneven Table: A Practical Approach to Dealing With Difference & Diversity (Kritek, 1996)

The Smart Woman's Guide to Interviewing and Salary Negotiation (King, 1995)

Negotiating for Your Life: New Success Strategies for Women (Schapiro, 1993)

Negotiation: Strategies for Mutual Gain (Hall, 1992)

Getting to Yes: Negotiating Agreement Without Giving In (Fisher & Ury, 1981)

Diagnose Yourself

1. Are you concerned about the finding that women physician faculty with children report lower career satisfaction (compared with men and with women without children)?

2. Do you think you have more or fewer role models with regard to leadership skills and professional development than your male peers?

3. Have you ever noticed that men are most comfortable with you when you smile and defer than when you express opinions differing from theirs? How do you handle this?

4. Have you ever experienced a conflict between being feminine and being competent? Have you ever been negatively labeled for behavior that is applauded in a man? How have you handled this?

5. How will you go about setting realistic career goals for yourself, given how quickly medicine is changing these days?

6. How might you apply the "PMI" exercise (plus, minus, interesting) to a choice you are considering?

7. Have you tried applying the "COPE" criteria to an analysis of your current commitments? Have you sought feedback on your outline from a trusted friend?

8. Have you tried practicing only starting sentences with "I" when they are about you? Are you "trimming hedges," (e.g., eliminating "I guess" unless it is really called for)?

9. Do you carry yourself with a "posture of power?"

10. What's an easy way to relax your whole body?

11. What are the five main conflict-management modes? Which ones do you most need to practice?

**Mentors:
Overcoming the
Shortage**

> When the student is ready, the teacher arrives.
> —*Ancient saying*

> When you see a turtle on the top of a fence, you can be sure she did not get there by herself.
> —*New saying*

Currently hailed in self-help publications as a "hot business fashion," the mentor concept is ancient. Mentor in Greek mythology was the teacher of Telemachus, son of Odysseus, who was off being a hero in the Trojan War. Less well-known is that Mentor was actually Athena, the Goddess of Wisdom, in disguise. (Perhaps Athena figured that Telemachus would better attend to her teachings coming from an older man; yes, even goddesses have to work at getting males to pay the right kind of attention!)

Odysseus intended Mentor to be a parent-substitute, but few young professionals today are seeking that level of supervision. Actually women in the professions are helping to update and reconceptualize mentoring. Some contrasts between the "old" and "new" ways: mentoring now is more about commitment between protégés and mentors than about chemistry, more about learning than power, more about personal growth and development than promotions and plums. Also, now protégés are more likely to pick their mentors than to wait passively for a senior person to select and "groom" them. This shift places much more responsibility on the protégé to assess her own goals and skill development needs.

The following pages provide many tips on obtaining and managing the mentoring you need and on maximizing the value of all your developmental relationships.

Why Women Still Miss Out

One of the first things women and minority students notice when they start medical school (if not college) is that entering students are highly diverse, but most faculty are white men. The homogeneity of the faculty contrasts sharply with the heterogeneity of the students and not just in terms of gender and ethnicity; there are other types of "nontraditional" student as well, such as students who are openly gay, who are from economically deprived backgrounds, who have been business executives. Almost all "nontraditional" students have a harder time finding mentors than those most resembling the majority of the faculty.

Most of the current generation of senior physicians evolved during an era when medicine was an apprenticeship. This one-on-one teaching model was taken for granted. Now that class sizes can number 200 and the complexities of medicine are so great, obviously this model is no longer operable. But because a new model of mentoring has not yet been developed, the needs of some young persons in medicine remain unmet.

Having a mentor is understood to be the most effective way to acquire an understanding of all the "unwritten rules" of succeeding along most career paths. For instance, one recent study showed that medical school faculty with a mentor reported greater career satisfaction than those without (Palepu et al., 1996). Another study found that women surgeons with a mentor worked significantly more hours (64/week) than those without (58/week) and published almost twice as many papers (7.5 vs. 4.7) (Neumayer, Levinson, & Putnam, 1995).

But women students, housestaff, and faculty do find fewer mentors and role models than men do (Haapanen, Ellsbury, & Schaad, 1996; Osborn et al., 1992). Even when they do find mentors, women are less likely to benefit from the relationship. For instance, compared with their male colleagues, women cardiologists found their mentors to be less helpful with career planning; and more than twice as many noted that their mentor was actually a negative role model (Limacher et al., 1998).

Women and minorities tend to be less assertive when approaching potential mentors or asking for what they need from mentors. This undermentoring has serious consequences because women actually have a greater need for mentoring than men do. Society still comparatively undervalues women's work and careers. Moreover, because women tend to underestimate their strengths more than men, they need extra help in learning to think positively and strategically about their careers and to garner the necessary resources (Jeruchim & Shapiro, 1992; Sandler et al., 1996).

Why is it harder for women than men to identify and make the best use of mentors? Think of mentoring as a dynamic reciprocal relationship with someone more advanced whom you respect. Many women have trouble finding both the "reciprocal" and "respect" aspects. Many women have trouble finding a male physician who combines all the qualities they want to emulate, particularly devotion to family. Also women's developmental stages are more complex than men's (i.e., their careers are less likely to proceed incrementally upward). Because of this extra complexity, many men are unable to identify fully with women protégés. Some men (especially those who have been falsely accused of sexual harassment) may avoid mentoring women to eliminate the hazards of intimacy issues or accusations. Moreover, because women are newer to the profession, some men understandably believe that mentoring a woman entails an increased risk of failure.

Naturally, women who prefer a woman mentor have fewer from whom to choose. Compared with the number of men physicians available as mentors, especially in surgery and most subspecialties, there are few women. Even in obstetrics and gynecology, where over 60% of residents are women, men (26,559) still far outnumber women practitioners (11,865) (American Medical Association, 1996). And because women physicians tend to have many other commitments laying claim to their energies, most are unable to spend as much time as they would like in mentoring young professionals. Women also tend to report feeling less qualified to be a mentor than men (Ragins & Cotton, 1993). As a self-fulfilling prophecy, women faculty ask "How can I be a good mentor when I never had one?"

Women who are ethnic minorities face even greater challenges to finding the mentoring they would consider optimal. For instance, at most schools black women medical students and faculty continue to be rare. Just in terms of overcoming feelings of isolation, though a black woman might prefer a mentor from a similar culture, she may have little success in identifying one. Even if she does find a black woman faculty member with whom she feels comfortable, that faculty member is probably already carrying way more than her weight in mentoring (and committee and other institutional) responsibilities. These extra responsibilities might be considered "affirmative abuse syndrome," that is the tendency of schools to overload their few minority faculty. Unfortunately, although intentions may be positive ("we need an African American on the curriculum committee"), the faculty member's own career progress is continually jeopardized; and the self-fulfilling prophecy is fulfilled. The result is very few minorities in leadership positions and very few role models for minority students.

In the mentor relationship, because of the gap between the senior and the junior person's level of power and authority, a great many things can go wrong as is evident from the Nine Circles of Mentor Hell (Figure 5.1). As an example of "overprotection," a study in one internal medicine department found that male mentors more actively promoted their men than their women mentees' participation in professional activities outside the institution (Fried et al., 1996). Because such participation is key to career success, these women were handicapped. This study also found a gender difference in the problem of "honorary authorship": Three times as many women as men protégés reported that their mentor utilized their work to advance the mentor's career rather than their own.

Another possible problem area in male-female mentoring dyads is a tendency for some men to relate to women more in terms of their social roles (e.g., father-daughter, husband-wife) than as professionals. A kind of unconscious paternalism can occur if a young woman reminds a man of his daughter; he may treat her very warmly, but without being aware of it, overprotect her or not push her as much as would be good for her. Moreover, men who have been taken care of all their lives by a mother and then a stay-at-home wife may expect deferential behavior from all women. If a female protégé challenges their advice, they may be insulted by what they perceive as her insubordination and lack of gratitude; with a male protégé, the challenge is more likely to be worked through rather than viewed as a threat to the relationship.

In addition to the above disadvantages, there are other reasons why women tend to underutilize professional relationships. Most women are accustomed to thinking of relationships in terms of support and affiliation, whereas men are accustomed to competition and hierarchy—more accurate descriptors for relationships in professional education and the workplace (see Chapter 4). Specifically women more than men medical students seek "kindness" and "approachability" in a mentor (Haapanen et al., 1996). Because these qualities

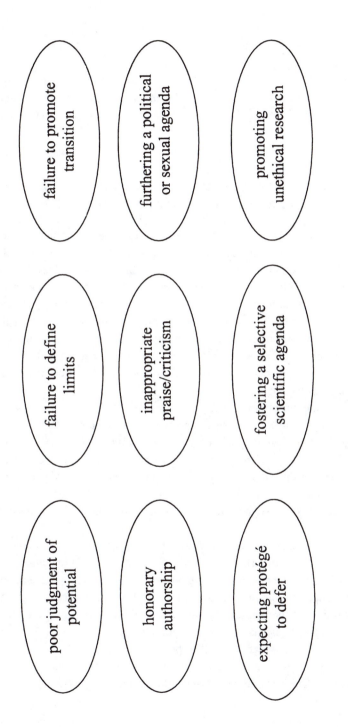

Figure 5.1. Nine Circles of Mentor Hell

are hard to find in busy faculty, it is no wonder women students are disappointed.

Do not be dismayed, however. Every year, more and more women physicians become available as mentors. And many men, especially secure, stable and happy ones, are great at mentoring women and want to get even better. It is up to you to find them and to avoid the pitfalls.

Finding and Using a Mentor: Avoiding the Nine Circles of Mentor Hell

There are many ways to conceptualize mentoring. The "godfather" model is the traditional one, a senior person looks for a younger version of himself to anoint. (Remember: "god*mothers*" only exist in fairy tales.) In this model, the mentor usually chooses the protégé, and much of the information exchange occurs in restaurants and golf courses. A more realistic model now is "it takes a village," with protégés choosing multiple mentors over the course of their careers because you will need very different types of support and challenge at different stages of your development. The advice below pertains mainly to the "multiple mentor" model, but most of the principles and cautions apply to all mentoring relationships.

Effective mentor/protégé interactions balance three key elements: support, challenge, and a vision of the protégé's future career (Bower, Diehr, Morzinski, & Simpson, 1998). Support refers to activities that affirm the value of the individual (e.g., displays of respect) and reduce anxiety (e.g., set clear expectations). While supporting their protégés, good mentors also challenge them to approach situations in new ways and point out inconsistencies in their actions and thinking. Mentors foster vision by stimulating discussions of the future.

As additional background, consider the progress of the levels of mentor involvement in the relationship. At the first level, "teaching," the mentor transfers knowledge to the mentee; the major investment is time. At the next level, "personal support," the mentor also offers motivation, direction, and confidence-building to the mentee. At the third level, "intervention," the mentor protects and helps advance the mentee, provides access to resources and may even forego relationships with other potential mentees. At the highest or "sponsorship" level, the mentor sponsors the mentee for otherwise unavailable opportunities. The higher the level, the more the mentor risks on behalf of the mentee (Andrew, 1996).

In addition to levels of involvement, the relationship can also be considered in terms of levels of imbalance. At the first level, the mentor is very directive and tells the mentee what to do and how to do it. At the next level, the mentor acknowledges the mentee's competencies and experience. At the third level, the mentor facilitates more give and take in the relationship. Finally, the mentee is ready for a lot of independence, and the mentor expects the mentee to contribute substantial information and value to exchanges.

Besides the information protégés contribute as the relationship progresses, mentors benefit in other ways. The relationship offers the mentor the satisfaction of assisting a junior colleague, the stimulation of time spent with a creative and energetic young person, bridges to future colleagues, the opportunity to practice managerial skills, and possible assistance with and collaborations on publications and grants.

What can you reasonably expect from a mentor? In approximate order from "immediately" to "when you have known each other awhile" expect the following:

- Advice on improving your clinical and teaching skills
- Advice on identifying and applying for grants and manuscript preparation
- Evaluating your strengths and weaknesses in a confidence-building way
- Identifying your talents and encouraging their development, especially through participation in organizations
- Advice on serving on committees, managing administrative responsibilities and negotiating institutional politics
- Help creating a personal "career vision," setting short- and long-term career goals and identifying opportunities
- Introductions to local and national experts in your specialty

If you are pursuing research, especially in a combined MD-PhD program, you will have a "built-in" mentor in your thesis adviser, laboratory director, or both. Research mentors play an especially important role in addition to the previously mentioned functions.

Here is a tested plan on how to approach a potential mentor:

- Start with as thorough a self-assessment as you can muster to gain clarity about your professional and personal goals and your immediate and projected skill development needs (see "Goal Setting" in Chapter 4).

- Depending on your comfort level and the person's location and accessibility, contact a potential mentor via snail-mail or e-mail with a brief proposal or request. Mention the qualities you admire about this person, and explain why these are important to you and how you want to gain from this person's insight and wisdom. Ask if the person can spare time for an initial interview.
- During the first contact, be brief and to the point, and try to keep an open mind and relaxed body.
- Follow up. Write a brief letter of appreciation, commenting on positive aspects of your meeting.
- Keep going down the list. If your first choice turns you down, try to find out why and be thankful for whatever you have learned. You will learn from each encounter.

Some additional advice gleaned from the experience of many young professionals follows:

- When you are reluctant to try something new, ask yourself (or have your mentor ask you) the following: "What is the worst thing that might happen?" "What is my (your) reluctance teaching me (you)?" "What will it take for me (you) to try this?"
- Be clear on what you have to give to the relationship; be your own best advocate but be realistic.
- Keep all scheduled appointments and dress appropriately.
- Be selective in what you absorb from a mentor, taking into account the person's values and character. Women sometimes feel dishonest if they do not embrace the whole character of the mentor; do not try to emulate what does not seem right to you.
- When seeking consultation, remember that the adviser may be giving you a recipe for the 1970s rather than for today or tomorrow.
- Maintain regular contact with mentors; the frequency will vary also depending on both of you—just do not lose touch completely.
- Nothing violates trust in a mentoring relationship faster than a breach of confidence. After all, the mentor has endeavored to give you an "inside" view and "thinks out loud" with you; hence you must respect this privilege or certainly risk losing it.
- Remember that despite all your precautions and plans, you will make mistakes. Accept your mistakes as your most memorable mentors (instead of repeatedly dragging yourself through the dirt of guilt and regret), and you will be well on your way not only to mental health but also success!

Finally, some extra cautions for women protégés to keep the relationship from becoming "toxic" include the following:

- Beware of overreliance or enmeshment, where a mentee adopts a mentor to the exclusion of other potentially helpful relationships.

- Boundary violations are common in any situation where there is vastly unequal power between the parties, especially in mixed gender mentoring. For instance, a male mentor may send out the following message to a young woman protégé: "I'll take care of you if you take care of my ego."

- Take care that the relationship does not become intimate, or even give the appearance of intimacy. Do not agree to meet in a bar or hotel room.

- If there is a cultural or gender difference between you and your mentor, you will probably need to actively discuss it. Try introducing the subject in a positive vein: share some information about your background and ask questions about your mentor's background. This can prevent erroneous assumptions and offer perspectives about your differences, so that respect rather than tension can build.

- In women more than men, seeking wise counsel may be interpreted as a sign of weakness. Therefore, be careful how you frame your request (e.g., rather than confessing "I must be really stupid, but," say, "I have this issue I'm trying to think through" or "I'm really impressed by how you led us through that agenda, would you be willing to help me understand how you managed that?"). If the answer is "no," do not apologize or feel personally rejected. The person just may not have the time to give you right now.

Thinking Institutionally

Medical student bodies are highly heterogeneous compared with the still largely white male faculty, and these new demographics challenge faculty in their establishing effective mentoring relationships. Moreover, as clinical pressures on faculty increase and funded time for academic endeavors decreases, conditions at academic medical centers are now less conducive to the mentoring of students, residents and junior faculty. Most faculty evaluation and reward mechanisms actually translate into disincentives for teaching and mentoring. The hard truth is that time spent with students does not generate income. (Tuition, however high, covers only a small fraction of the costs of running a medical school.)

One institutional improvement is to include the following dimensions of mentoring on students' evaluations of faculty at the end of each course and clerkship:

- Demonstrates respectful attitude toward my work
- Provides timely feedback
- Gives constructive feedback on skills
- Gives counsel on important professional decisions
- Provides guidance on professional ethics

Over time, students' ratings of faculty on these dimensions would create a database on each faculty members' dedication to the professional development of trainees that could be considered in promotion decisions.

This is just one idea among many to build more institutional support for mentoring. Many schools, usually via the Women in Medicine program or organized by an energetic group of women students, publish lists of faculty who wish to mentor students or a directory of women faculty. A few medical schools have started mentoring programs for students. Perhaps the best organized is Case Western Reserve University's Mentoring Advisor Program, created by the Office of Student Affairs. A few medical schools, most notably the University of Arkansas and Stanford University, have also created mentoring programs that help to pair junior women faculty with volunteering senior faculty.

Medical schools are increasingly becoming more cost and energy conscious and are seeing that the "trial and error method" of career development wastes time and talent. So many benefits accrue to the institution when the next generation is being well-mentored. Strong mentoring relationships increase the stability and health of the institution, contribute to a climate of cooperation, increase faculty and student satisfaction, enhance the career development of women and minorities, and develop future leaders.

Building Your Network

Because of the rapid change in medicine and competition for the best mentors, it is expedient to consider Mentor Replacement Therapy (and well before you need Hormone Replacement Therapy!). From the very outset of your education as a professional, look for opportunities to expand your network of col-

TABLE 5.1 Developmental Relationships

Career Functions	Psychosocial Functions
Sponsorship: opening doors	Role modeling
Coaching: teaching; providing feedback	Counseling
Protection: providing support; acting as buffer	Acceptance and confirmation
Exposure: creating opportunities	Friendship
Challenge: providing "stretch" assignments	

leagues. Even if you have a mentor, it is useful to think in terms of a continuum of collegial relationships—individuals you can look to as coach, guide, advocate, role model, or advisor for different purposes and at different times.

For instance, you might meet a student at the American Medical Student Association national convention who shares your interest in creating a student-staffed preventive health clinic. You decide to write a grant together but neither of you knows how to go about this. You attend the handy workshop at the convention on grant-writing and decide to ask the leader (who happens to be an assistant professor at your new friend's school) to help you get started, and she agrees to read your first draft and to share some additional materials with you, as she is also interested in this research. You might consider her a "topic" mentor, and you might consider your threesome "short-term learning partners" for purposes of this project. This relationship may be time-limited or may evolve into an even more significant professional relationship down the line.

Without becoming too utilitarian about it, you should always be thinking about expanding your network of developmental relationships. Developmental relationships serve many functions, both career-wise and psychosocially (see Table 5.1). Do you currently have a developmental relationship with someone you respect

- Who is ethical and can keep a confidence?
- Who respects your values, gender, culture and ethnicity?
- Who is willing to provide support and help you resolve personal problems?
- Who you consider a role model and who will give you objective advice, even if it stings?

As with more formal mentoring relationships, minorities of all kinds face extra challenges in forming developmental relationships. Here are a few of the reasons:

- Relationships occur most naturally between "like" individuals who are very "comfortable" with each other (why men and women are often most relaxed in single-sex groups). Are you more comfortable with role models who "look like you"?
- Majority individuals are seldom able to fully empathize with minorities.
- The performance of minorities is scrutinized more closely and problems remembered for disproportionate lengths of time.
- Society still undervalues women's intellectual work compared with men's.
- Women face higher hurdles to prove themselves to potential mentors.
- Young women sometimes feel "personally betrayed" if a senior woman is not helpful, holding the senior women to higher standards than they hold men (see Chapter 3).

Unrelated to gender or ethnic factors, some people simply need help in developing their "mentor receptors" (Grady-Weliky, Kettyle, & Hundert, in press). They need to be taught about the need for mentoring and for introducing themselves and forming networks. If this sounds familiar, the following points will be useful:

- Realize that you can learn from every person—from bad as well as good examples.
- Create a "support-listen-respond system." Ask a trusted colleague to play the devil's advocate with you to challenge your unspoken assumptions, assess your skills and deficiencies, and provoke you to consider alternatives.
- Do not be afraid to initiate conversations with individuals you respect. For example, introduce yourself to a speaker at a meeting if there is an overlap of interests. Most people enjoy receiving praise and being sought after for their expertise.
- Learn from observing the successful networking of others.

Diagnose Yourself

1. What does Athena, the Goddess of Wisdom, have to do with the origin of the concept of mentoring?
2. Why do women tend to have even greater mentoring needs than men?

3. Why might you anticipate greater difficulties than your male peers in identifying and making the best use of mentors?

4. How do you approach a potential mentor? What if your first choice turns you down?

5. Name a few of the nine circles of mentor hell. How do you plan to avoid them?

6. What can you reasonably expect from a physician who has agreed to be your mentor?

7. What are proactive steps you can take to prevent misunderstandings with your mentor related to differences in your gender and cultural background?

8. Have "boundary violations" in a relationship ever been a problem for you (i.e., allowing someone to become too dependent on you or vice versa)? If so, how will you prevent this from occurring with your mentor?

9. How will you go about building your network of professional colleagues?

6 Big Hairy Questions (BHQs): Into the Future

The future belongs to those who believe in the beauty of their dreams.
—*Eleanor Roosevelt*

The previous chapters have grounded you in current realities for women in medicine and offered guides to maximizing your options. Undoubtedly you still have some Big Hairy Questions (BHQs) about how you and a medical career intersect. Here are a few additional perspectives to help you look and plan ahead. If your particular BHQ is not addressed, one of the Websites included in Appendix F might help. The only constant these days is accelerating change. Questions will always outnumber answers. So hang loose. And remember the poet Rainer Maria Rilke's advice: "Have patience with all that is unresolved in your heart and try to love the questions themselves."

When I Complete My Training, Will I Be Able to Find a Job?

As a profession, medicine is being buffeted as never before by powerful forces that are changing it in fundamental ways. Among these forces are (a) pressures to control costs while improving the quality of care; (b) the explosion of genetic and scientific knowledge of enormous potential benefit, increasing patient expectations that their physicians be both "hi-tech" and "hi-touch"; and (c) the computer and Internet revolutions' transforming effects on the amount of information available to both providers and consumers.

At the same time, because of the "new health care team," physicians face more competition (Carlson, 1999). An array of health care workers less highly paid than physicians (e.g., nurse practitioners) are now providing services formerly handled only by physicians. More and more Americans are seeking care from "alternative" providers such as acupuncturists and massage therapists. Moreover, a few areas of the country are becoming saturated with physicians. Thus, questions about job possibilities and security (that were nonissues a generation ago) are now on the minds of many physicians and medical school applicants. Applicants will likely get a different answer from each physician they ask about these issues, because there is so much variability from place to place, specialty to specialty—and some physicians are much more adaptable than others.

Only one recent study sheds reliable light here. Physicians completing residencies in May 1996 were surveyed about their experiences securing a job beginning that year. By November over 12,000 (48%) had responded; and of these only 7% had not found a position. Of those who found a position, 22% reported significant difficulty in finding one. Those reporting the most difficulty were international medical school graduates (i.e., from non-U.S. schools), those completing programs in the Pacific or north central region, and those in anesthesiology, gastroenterology, infectious disease, pulmonary, ophthalmology, pathology, plastic surgery and radiology. Male physicians (26%) reported more difficulty than female physicians (17%) finding positions; there was no gender difference in the number of job offers received (Miller, Dunn, Richter, & Whitcomb, 1998).

Although cautionary, the results of this major study need to be interpreted in context, that is, individuals completing other types of graduate and professional degree programs also face challenges landing a desirable job. Over 90% of those finishing a residency in 1996 had found a job within months of completion of their training. Plus the large majority of these new physicians reported no difficulty finding a position, and women were significantly less likely to report difficulty than men.

What Does It Take to Be a Success in Medicine?

This question is harder to answer now than in previous eras. In prior decades, if you graduated from a U.S. medical school and completed residency, you were virtually assured of earning a good living and finding desirable opportunities.

But even in those less complicated times, did all these physicians consider themselves "successful"? That is impossible to answer. Now with more constraints and complexities, medical careers—even established ones—are flapping in the winds of change. The experience of previous generations of physicians ("bygone docs") will not provide a roadmap. Managed care necessitates more managed careers. Apply a prevention and fitness model, including push-ups (i.e., hard work) and periodic "check-ups" with an up-to-date mentor or trainer.

Physicians who provide career counseling to burned out or otherwise disoriented physicians offer these "new rules" for physicians' careers:

- Most physicians need to acquire many skills not covered in medical education. Such skills include learning to (a) challenge assumptions about yourself and your career (heeding Mark Twain's words: "What I don't know is not as much of a problem as what I am sure I know that just ain't so"), (b) work with a diverse and empowered team without being "in charge," and (c) understand cash flow and financial statements (Haid, 1998). You might consider a joint MD-Master's of Business Administration (MBA) program or a complementary MBA program designed specifically for physicians. Examples of the latter include the following:

  – University of Houston, Clear Lake, School of Business and Public Administration's MBA Program for Physicians
  – University of California, Irvine, Graduate School of Management's Health Care Executive MBA Program
  – University of South Florida College of Business Administration's MBA for Physicians Program
  – University of Tennessee, Knoxville, College of Business Administration's Physician Executive MBA

- Adaptability is a key asset.
- Information is power. Acquire basic computer skills, including use of e-mail and the Internet as efficient vehicles for exchanging and gaining information. Read outside your field.
- Build a diverse professional network (see Chapter 5).
- Even if you work for a large organization, consider yourself "self-employed," that is, responsible for your own career development.

- Do not allow your career to fully define you (women do not tend to fall into this trap as often as men).

Try to think in the "future tense." What does our society increasingly need? Most believe we need more physicians skilled in complementary (also called alternative or integrative) medicine, geriatrics, behavior modification, and telemedicine and who are both patient advocates and community health advocates, and who understand accountability, information management, and epidemiology.

What About Becoming a Medical School Faculty Member?

Do you enjoy teaching and being in an environment where there is active inquiry and the next generation is always asking questions? Do you hope to help shape the future of medicine? If yes, you probably won't be happy unless you remain in an academic medical center. There are many ways of combining the practice of medicine with academic pursuits, including as a volunteer faculty, as a full-time practitioner with a part-time paid faculty appointment, and as a full-time academic who combines clinical, research, teaching and administrative responsibilities with a medical school or teaching hospital as the primary employer.

In addition to "being where the action is," other benefits of an academic appointment are topnotch, easy access to information resources and receiving a regular paycheck without either the responsibilities of running a business or the strictures attendant to working for a managed care organization.

Prospective academics especially benefit from early career planning. Writing grants and securing research funding take time and require the help of mentors. If you enjoy research or think you might, do not delay in exploring this route—opportunity abounds at most academic medical centers.

A few words about finding a research niche. Basic biomedical research in a scientific laboratory is far from the only possibility. Your "laboratory" can also be the hospital, the classroom, an ambulatory clinic, the health system, or the community. Scholarly inquiry can and needs to be conducted by physicians in all these settings.

If you are happiest working in an environment where there is active inquiry and where you can affect the future health care of many, an academic career, with its additional challenges and benefits, is probably for you.

Are Men and Women Physicians Becoming More Alike or Different?

In 1980, 11% of U.S. physicians were women; by 1996, this proportion doubled to 22%. Now, 43% of medical students are women (see Appendix B). It is impossible to predict at what point this proportion will top out. In the meantime, questions arise about whether differences between men and women physicians are increasing or decreasing, and whether women are in a better or worse position to thrive in the changing world of medicine.

Naturally most men get defensive when anyone asks whether women make better doctors. Most studies do find that women physicians are more likely to provide more "patient centered" and empathic care than men (Bertakis, Helms, Callahan, Azari, & Robbins, 1995; Brooks, 1998). They spend more time in direct communication with patients, listening and in more collaborative exchanges, facilitating a greater degree of continuity of care (Morantz-Sanchez, 1994). Women physicians also discuss prevention of illness and family issues more frequently (Bertakis et al., 1995; Lurie et al., 1993). These "nurturing" qualities are certainly beneficial to patients. No wonder women physicians are sued less often than men.

If you are practicing in a setting with preset patient visit quotas, the proclivity to spend more time with each patient can become a stress (Andrew & Bickel, 1998). In a recent study of primary care physicians, women physicians reported more negative effects of managed care; it impaired the time available per patient, the physician-patient relationship, and quality of care (Feldman, Novack, & Gracely, 1998). Similarly, a study of women general practitioners in Britain found the sample felt especially stressed by demands to be sensitive and caring while working within an environment where the dominant values are clinical objectivity and professional distance (Brooks, 1998).

Some patients expect that women physicians will be more caring than men physicians and hold them to a higher standard of caring, which may lead to unfortunate disappointments. Men and women patients can present different challenges. In one recent study, patients of both genders were least satisfied with younger physicians, especially male patients with younger female physicians. This devaluation may stem from old ideas about what a "physician should look like" (Hall, Irish, Roter, Ehrlich, & Miller, 1994). On the other hand, male patients responded more positively when female physicians introduced emotional or personal issues than when male physicians did.

Men physicians continue to log in more work hours, although the difference between men and women physicians' work weeks continues to steadily decrease. Although women do work fewer hours per week during their childbearing years, they live longer and practice to an older age. As women spend more time than men professionals engaged with their families, they tend to "interweave several tasks together, with issues of identity, generativity and intimacy revisited several times" (Kaltreider, 1997, p. 243). This undulating path is more natural, balanced, and healthy in the long run than a total career focus for the first couple decades and then early retirement due to poor health, with few hobbies, family or friends to enjoy during one's declining years.

Moreover, most women physicians are very healthy. The largest-ever study of women physicians has found that women physicians have better health habits than other socioeconomically advantaged women; their health-related behaviors exceed all national recommended standards (Frank, Brogan, Mokdad, et al., 1998).

To conclude on another positive note, the most recent studies show that women are now becoming board certified at the same rate as men—93% of young men and 92% of young women physicians (Xu, Veloski, & Hojat, 1998). Because specialty board certification is becoming a universal criterion for a license to practice and is prerequisite to hospital appointments and recruitment into a managed care organization, this high rate of certification is evidence of important progress from earlier eras.

Do Women Have More Unmet Health Care Needs Than Men?

Few would disagree that gender continues to structure life opportunities and changes, but is there a cost to being a woman with regard to health and health care (Hunt & Allandale, 1999)? Although women live longer than men, their longevity carries a greater lifetime risk of disability and chronic illness, including cancer, cardiovascular disease and dementia. Women receive fewer therapies of demonstrated effectiveness for a variety of conditions (Haas, 1998) and are more likely to have their symptoms attributed to psychiatric causes (Tobin et al., 1987). Overall, women tend to be less satisfied with their health care than men (Falik & Scott-Collins, 1996). In fact, care delivered to women has been described as "fragmented, incomplete and poorly coordinated" (Council on Graduate Medical Education, 1995). Older women see internists who may not perform necessary pap smears or breast examinations. Women of reproductive age may see only gynecologists who may not manage their health needs that are unrelated to their reproductive organs.

There are problems with insurance too. Women are less likely to have private health insurance because they are more likely to work part-time (Miles & Parker, 1997). Moreover, Medicare does not serve women as well as men as it provides less adequate coverage for nursing home care, community services, outpatient medications and preventive health maintenance (Miles & Parker).

On a positive note, it is increasingly understood that the health care needs of women do not begin and end with the uterus. Women's health is now incorporating all organ systems as well as mental health status and women's preferences for care (Haas, 1998; see Appendices D and E). Women's health research is now focusing on gender-based differences at the cellular and molecular level, across all life cycles, and on evidence of effectiveness of therapy (Marshall, 1997).

Will Women's Health
Become a Separate Specialty?

Since 1990 when Congress mandated inclusion of women in clinical trials and established the National Institutes of Health (NIH) Office of Research on Women's Health (ORWH), women's health has gained increasing attention among policymakers and physicians. The ORWH developed an agenda that set the stage for many other national initiatives to improve women's health care and education over the last decade. For instance, the U.S. Department of Health and Human Services (DHHS), Public Health Service (PHS) also established an Office on Women's Health (PHS-OWH) to coordinate a comprehensive women's health agenda within the DHHS (see Appendix F). Since 1996, the PHS-OWH has designated annually six national Centers of Excellence (COE) in women's health to serve as models for improving the health care of women.

In 1994 a group of physicians, medical educators, medical association staff and educators formed the National Academy on Women's Health Medical Education (NAWHME), initiated jointly by the MCP Hahnemann University School of Medicine and the American Medical Women's Association. A valuable product of NAWHME's work is *Women's Health in the Curricu-*

lum: A Resource Guide for Faculty which includes a practical definition of women's health (see Appendix E), a comprehensive list of women's health competencies, and a list with brief descriptions of women's health education programs.

The Association of Professors of Gynecology and Obstetrics (APGO) has also convened medical educators across disciplines and medical association representatives to create an interdisciplinary curriculum in women's health care. The resulting *Essential Learning Objectives in Women's Health* (1996; see Appendix D) outlines the knowledge, skills, and attitudes recommended for medical student competency in women's health. APGO next established a Women's Health Care Education Office to promote and coordinate an integrated, multidisciplinary approach to women's health care education. APGO and the Association of American Medical Colleges are also bringing together physicians and medical educators interested in fostering interdisciplinary women's health activities at medical schools and teaching hospitals.

Some activists suggest that for women's health to receive the prominence and funding it deserves, it needs to be a separate specialty. Critics say that insisting on "separateness" will result in marginalization of women's health. Moreover, separating "women's" from "men's" health is all but impossible because differentiating between the sexes is not always clear-cut. More importantly, by definition women's health is multidisciplinary.

To be sure, the interdisciplinary nature of women's health adds a level of difficulty to its integration into medical school curricula, because curricular change has traditionally followed an "add and/or substitute" strategy (Nelson, Nicolete, & Johnson, 1997). A better approach would be to add segments to existing courses or to create new interdisciplinary courses (Jonassen et al., 1999; Kwolek, Griffith, & Blue, 1999).

Just in the last few years, a variety of materials have been published to support medical education's increasing focus on women's health and to serve as resources to laypersons and physicians. Some of the best books include the following:

- *Textbook of Women's Health* (Wallis, 1998)
- *A New Prescription for Women's Health: Getting the Best Medical Care in a Man's World* (Healy, 1995)
- *The Women's Complete Healthbook* (Epps & Stewart, 1995)
- *Women's Primary Health Care: Office Practice and Procedures* (Seltzer & Pearse, 1995)

Appendix A
Foremothers

People . . . ask not, Is she capable, but, Is this fearfully capable person nice? Will she upset our ideal of womanhood and maidenhood, and the social relations of the sexes? Can a woman physician be lovable; can she marry; can she have children; will she take care of them? If she cannot, what is she?

—*Mary Putnam Jacobi, Shall Women Practice Medicine?*
(1882; quoted in Lovejoy, 1957, p. 10).

When it comes to women as physicians, "We've come a long way, baby!" To put the challenges women have faced into perspective, until a century ago, a woman's identity was based largely on her relationship to men. As society moved from an agricultural to an industrial base in the mid-19th century, a woman's sphere broadened but remained based in domesticity as homemaker and family and child care provider (Tom, 1997). Although women did gain a leadership role privately in the home, publicly they were allowed only a subordinate role. The questions posed by Dr. Jacobi in the opening quotation remained all too real.

Even though women's focus on the family positioned them to fight for health and social causes, women who practiced medicine in the 19th century were met with shock (Tom, 1997). Women doctors had to function in a society that was structured around men, most of whom resented female deviance from traditional roles. Even women considered women doctors more like "grannies" than serious doctors (Luchetti, 1998). Moreover, women were considered unfit to practice because of "the physical and mental disturbances induced by menstruation" (Roth Walsh, 1977). Consequently, up until the current century, even though they provided a great deal of care, women remained peripheral to mainstream medicine, serving either as midwives or in subordinate roles as nurses. Those few who did practice as physicians were not allowed access to the same medical training as men.

Seventeen women's medical colleges opened in the United States between 1848 and 1900; five of these later merged with male-only institutions and nine did not survive into the 20th century. By 1900, over 1,200 women were enrolled in U.S. medical colleges and over 7,000 women physicians were in practice (Roth Walsh, 1977). But beginning in 1910, curricular standardization and the advent of physician licensing requirements added rigor heretofore missing from U.S. medical education. Of the 17 women's medical colleges, only the Women's Medical College of Pennsylvania remained open after Abraham Flexner's Report and investigations, thus acting to decrease women's access to a medical education.

But throughout these years, women never stopped trying to gain access to mainstream medicine. For instance, Dr. Harriot Hunt had already practiced medicine for 12 years when she applied to Harvard; she was rejected twice. After a donor promised a gift on condition of Harvard's admission of women, Hunt was grudgingly enrolled (but never granted a degree). Male students protested her presence: "No woman of true delicacy would be willing in the presence of men to listen to medical discussions" (Luchetti, 1998). Similarly, in 1882 a group of prominent Boston women physicians offered Harvard $50,000 with the stipulation that its medical school open admissions to women; again the offer was rejected. (Harvard did not admit women medical students until 1945.) Johns Hopkins University set a precedent by opening its doors to women medical students in 1893, after a group of women benefactors offered $500,000 to the medical school if women were admitted on the same terms as men.

When World Wars I and II cut the supply of male medical school applicants and staff physicians, many male-only institutions opened admissions to women. However, after the wars, just as they told "Rosie the Riveter" to go home, practicing women physicians were also removed from staff and clinic positions to make room for returning veterans.

The largest leap in the number of female medical school applicants occurred during the first half of the 1970s, when their numbers nearly quadrupled, rising from under 2,300 to just over 8,700. By 1975, women were over 20% of the total applicant pool. Several forces were at work during the 1970s, beginning with an overall change in women's aspirations engendered by the "consciousness raising" of the feminist movement. Also important was the passage of Title IX of the Civil Rights Act of 1972, which stated that no person would, on the basis of sex, be excluded from participation in, be denied the benefits of, or be subjected to discrimination under any education program receiving federal assistance.

This highly abbreviated history of the long way we've come can in no way convey the courage of those first pioneering women physicians. Here are a few of the most stellar of your "foremoms":

- Probably the first English-speaking woman physician was Dr. James Miranda Barry, who served as a medical officer and inspector-general of the British Army hospitals between 1813 and 1865. She was found to have been a woman only after her death (Lovejoy, 1957).

- Elizabeth Blackwell was the first woman graduate of a U.S. medical school, Geneva Medical College in New York in 1849, where she was also first in her class. She was shunned by fellow students and the community and also excluded from clinical demonstrations. Provoked by these early obstacles, she went on to establish, in 1868, one of the first women's medical colleges, the Women's Medical College of New York Infirmary. She also set up a free clinic, The New York Infirmary for Indigent Women and Children, now known as the New York Infirmary/ Beekman Downtown Hospital (Weisman, 1998).

- Former faculty member of the New England Female Medical College and protégé of Elizabeth Blackwell, Marie Zakrzewska founded the New England Hospital for Women and Children. Owned and operated by women, the Hospital provided internship training denied to women by most hospitals.

- Nancy Talbot Clark was the first woman physician in the United States to seek certification from a state medical society (1852).

- In 1864, Rebecca Lee was the first black woman to receive a medical degree in the United States.

- Dr. Mary Putnam Jacobi, who studied under Dr. Zakrzewska, gained notoriety for dispelling Harvard professor E. H. Clarke's theory that women's inferior biological status made them unsuitable for medical practice. Her essay, "The Question of Rest for Women During Menstruation," disproved Clarke's theory with statistical analyses and case studies (Morantz-Sanchez, 1985).

Appendix B
Statistical Overview

Applicants and Students

In 1998, the proportion of women in the U.S. medical school applicant pool stood at 43.3%. Compared to rapid growth in the 1970s and steady growth in the 1980s, the proportion of women applicants has plateaued. Recently, women have been accepted into medical school at a slightly higher rate than men. In 1998, women constituted 43% of new entrants and almost 43% of total enrollment in U.S. medical schools.

There are large school-to-school variations in the proportion of new entrants who are women, from a low in 1998 of 23% to a high of 63%. During the 1997 to 1998 academic year, women made up the majority of new entrants at 20 schools.

Residents

The proportion of women in residency programs has grown from 22% of all residents in 1980 to 35% in 1996 and 36% in 1997. The specialty with the highest proportion of women residents is pediatrics, where 64% are women, followed by obstetrics/gynecology with 63%. The proportion of women in most of the surgical subspecialties remains low: orthopedic surgery, 7%; urology, 10%; and thoracic surgery, 5%.

Of the 34,882 women residents in 1997, over one-quarter are training in internal medicine (including subspecialties). The next highest concentrations are 16% in pediatrics (including subspecialties), 14% in family practice, 9% in obstetrics/gynecology, and 7% in psychiatry (including child psychiatry). The proportion of all women residents who are training in each of the surgical subspecialties remains below 1% (e.g., neurosurgery, plastic surgery, and urology garner less than .4% each; thoracic surgery and colon/rectal, less than .1% of all women residents).

Medical School Faculty

The proportion of full-time faculty who are women was 26% in 1998, totaling 22,970. Orthopedic surgery continues to have the lowest proportion of faculty who are women (9%), and pediatrics, the highest (40%).

Clinical departments that have seen the greatest increases in the representation of women since 1989 are emergency medicine (1.8 times, from 13% to 23%), ophthalmology (1.6 times, from 14% to 23%), OB/GYN (1.6 times, from 24% to 38%), family practice (1.6 times, from 24% to 34%), dermatology (1.5 times, from 21% to 32%), and internal medicine (1.5 times, from 16% to 24%).

The departments where the highest proportions of full professors are women are public health (19%), anatomy (18%), pediatrics (18%), and microbiology (16%). In orthopedic surgery, only 2% of full professors are women. The number of women full professors is growing very slowly. Between 1997 and 1998, the number of women basic science professors grew from 811 to 834, and in clinical sciences from 1,493 to 1,533.

Of all women faculty, just above 10% are full professors; 19% are associate professors; 50% are assistant professors; 17% are instructors. Men are much more evenly distributed across professional ranks—31%, 25%, 35%, and 8%, respectively. These distributions across the ranks have not changed for men or women in over 15 years.

On average there are 19 women full professors per medical school including nontenured and basic sciences faculty, compared to 160 men full professors per school.

With regard to the ethnic breakdown of women faculty, 18% are not Caucasian. Compared to Caucasian faculty, underrepresented minority groups have higher proportions of women faculty.

Medical School Deans

In 1998, nine of the 125 U.S. medical school deans were women—Dr. Bernadine Healy, Ohio State University College of Medicine; Dr. Amira Gohara, Medical College of Ohio; Dr. Patricia Monteleone, St. Louis University School of Medicine; Dr. Barbara Atkinson, MCP Hahnemann University School of Medicine; Dr. Julia Bonilla, Universidad Central del Caribe; Dr. Deborah Powell, University of Kansas School of Medicine; Dr. Marjorie Sirridge (interim), University of Missouri, Kansas City School of Medicine; Dr. Carolyn Robinowitz, Georgetown University School of Medicine; and Dr. Anna Cherrie Epps, Meharry Medical School (Bickel, Croft, & Marshall, 1998).

Appendix C
Addressing Gender Inequities and Sexism

Assessing Gender Fairness

To assess the equity of the environment for women at the University of Virginia School of Medicine, the Committee on Women surveyed all faculty, residents and students (Hostler & Gressard, 1993). Following are examples of items from the survey, with instructions: "Circle the response which best describes how you feel: strongly disagree, disagree, agree, strongly agree, not applicable/don't know."

- There is an atmosphere that enables women physicians and scientists to fully participate in teaching, administrative, and research activities.
- There tends to be a condescending attitude toward women physicians and scientists in the Medical Center.
- Men are more likely than women to receive helpful career advice from their supervisors.
- There is recognition of the presence and importance of women and their contributions on the wards and in the classroom.
- Women are adequately represented as visiting professors and invited speakers.
- Women are appropriately represented among the tenured faculty and in the senior administrative positions.

- There is an adequate number of female faculty as role models for students and housestaff.

- Sexist remarks are heard on rounds in the classroom.

Sexism Discussion Case

(To be adapted to stimulate discussion in courses on social and bioethical issues or during student orientation or workshops on gender issues)

Jane is a member of the first class at Prestige Medical School in which the proportion of women is over 50%. The faculty generally agrees that this class is one of the most energetic and committed in recent memory, but some are unprepared for and uncomfortable with this large a group of women. In turn many of the women notice that the 70 kilogram white male is presented as the standard to illustrate test results and clinical findings. By the end of the second year, Jane is notorious for asking faculty to detail significance and differences relative to female anatomy and physiology. Although some students of both sexes appreciate her efforts, a number of her classmates wish she would "give it a rest."

A new and highly regarded obstetrics and gynecology division chief gives a key lecture. Included in Dr. Blunt's slides are shots of female genitalia displayed in sexually suggestive ways. Jane interrupts the lecture, charging Dr. Blunt with treating women as if they were sexual objects. A number of men students hiss their disapproval at her interpretation and interruption. Jane walks out of the room and into the student dean's office, accompanied by a few other women. The student dean arranges a meeting between Dr. Blunt and the concerned students. Dr. Blunt explains that he had been showing those slides to students for years, with no complaints. When the students explain why they find the images offensive, he states that indeed part of his goal is to "desensitize" students to the potentially sexually arousing patients they would encounter. After a long discussion regarding how such "desensitization" might better be achieved, Dr. Blunt agrees not to use those slides again. However, he also makes it clear that he believes this handful of students is overreacting.

Jane has known for years that she wants to become an obstetrician/gynecologist and has eagerly awaited this rotation. But by the end of the fourth week of her OB/GYN clerkship, Jane is very uncomfortable. A couple of the residents regularly speak condescendingly to their patients, many of whom are African American. Jane can barely resist confronting these residents but restrains herself out of fear for her evaluation. Finally, after hearing a resident say in a loud voice to a crying woman "Honey, I just don't have time to explain the procedure right now," Jane runs after him, pointing out his lack of respect for this patient. He explodes at Jane that she doesn't know what she's talking about and that he is late for a meeting with Dr. Blunt.

During the last week of her clerkship, Jane overhears a conversation in a corridor between two of the women residents. One had just overheard Dr. Blunt say to a group of residents "None of my residents had better get pregnant. We run a tight ship here. I expect 100% from everyone." Jane asks them if they are going to respond to Dr. Blunt's "encroachment on their individual rights." They advise Jane to pipe down if she wants to get into an OB/GYN residency.

What should Jane do? Questions to probe this scenario follow:

1. What are students' responsibilities relative to faculty when they have a grievance or when they disagree with or disapprove of teaching methods or materials? What kind of process would be optimal in resolving such conflicts? Are there structures and resources for addressing continuing problems with sexism in medical education?

2. Does a student have a responsibility for action after witnessing a patient being treated in less than respectful ways? How can students resolve tensions they experience between being a "team player" versus a "truth-teller?" Does it matter whether the problem is with a nurse, a resident, an attending, or a department head? Because of their long hours and often difficult working conditions, should residents ever be excused for using humor at patients' expense?

3. The multiple missions of medical centers create a complex environment that is often far from optimal for student education. What problems with this OB/GYN clerkship most need to be addressed? Should students have the opportunity to rate faculty and residents on professional behaviors? What resources might help Jane with her bind between her conscience and the need for a good evaluation and good references?

Outline for a Medical Student Workshop or Elective on Gender Stereotypes

(These can be adapted by individual faculty and student groups.)
Possible workshop objectives include the following:

- Encourage women students to increase their valuing and use of an emphatic style and examine stereotypes of "feminine" and "masculine" styles

- Increase students' appreciation for the complexity of gendered experience
- Increase their reflection on their own experience and development and increase their valuing of self-reflection
- Facilitate students imagining a more humanistic practice of medicine.

Hypotheses to promote discussion on the experiences of medical students follow:

- Female medical students have conflicts about their visibility.
- Female medical students experience lack of support from family.
- Medical students struggle with the lack of a realistic ego-ideal.
- Males struggle with unrealistic expectations of omnipotence.
- Females struggle with combining the opposing constraints of both traditional feminine and traditional masculine roles.

Appendix D
Learning Objectives in Women's Health

The Association of Professors of Gynecology and Obstetrics (APGO; 1996) has developed knowledge and skill competencies in the following areas, recommending that all disciplines caring for women emphasize these. The competencies may be obtained from APGO (see Appendix F).

Autoimmune Diseases
Breast Disease
Cardiovascular Disease
Contraception, Sterilization, and Abortion
Diagnosis and Management Plan
Domestic Violence and Sexual Assault
Gastrointestinal Disorders
Gynecologic Malignancies
Immunizations
Maternal-Fetal Physiology
Menopause
Menstrual Cycle and Its Abnormalities
Nutrition
Papanicolaou Smear and Culture
Pelvic Pain
Pharmacology

Physical Exam
Preconception, Antepartum, and Postpartum
Premenstrual Syndrome
Psychiatric and Behavioral Problems
Pulmonary Disease
Sexuality
Sexually Transmitted Diseases
Spontaneous Abortion and Ectopic Pregnancy
Urinary Tract Disorders
Vulvar and Vaginal Diseases

Appendix E
Definition of Women's Health

Women's Health is devoted to facilitating the

- preservation of wellness and
- prevention of illness in women,

and includes screening, diagnosis, and management of conditions which

- are unique to women,
- are more common in women,
- are more serious in women, and
- have manifestations, risk factors, or interventions which are different in women.

Women's Health also recognizes and includes

- the importance of the study of gender differences,
- multidisciplinary team approaches,
- the values and knowledge of women and their own experience of health and illness,
- the diversity of women's health needs over the life cycle, and how these needs reflect differences in race, class, ethnicity, culture, sexual preference, levels of education, and access to medical care, and

- includes the empowerment of women, as for all patients, to be informed participants in their own health care (National Academy of Women's Health in Medical
  Education, 1996).

Appendix F
Organizations and Websites

It is not what you know, it's how fast you can find out.
—*Anonymous*

General Medical Organizations

Association of American Medical Colleges (AAMC): http://www.aamc.org; telephone: (202) 828-0400; AAMC Publications Office: telephone: (202) 828-0416. The AAMC is a nonprofit organization representing 125 medical schools in the United States and 16 in Canada, and approximately 400 teaching hospitals and 86 academic and professional societies. AAMC conducts a broad range of programs in the areas of medical education, biomedical research, health care for the nation, related policy issues, student and applicant relations, and more. Information on AAMC's Website especially valuable for medical students includes the following:

- Medical College Admission Test (MCAT)
- American Medical College Application Service (AMCAS), including a downloadable version of the AMCAS-E (electronic application) software
- MEDLOANS, a comprehensive loan program developed to provide financial assistance to medical students
- Organization of Student Representatives (OSR), student representation from each U.S. medical school as a principal voice and vehicle for enhancing medical education and academic medicine

- National Residency Matching Program (NRMP) and Electronic Residency Application Service (ERAS)

- AAMC's Community and Minority Programs, activities and resources to support and increase the number of underrepresented minority students in medical and other health professional schools

- AAMC's Women in Medicine Program, activities and resources to support women's advancement and leadership potential

- MedCAREERS, a career planning tool developed jointly by the AAMC and AMA, is available online at www.aamc.org/medcareers.

- AAMC sponsors a *Medical School Admission Requirements* electronic mailing list called MSAR_Clipboard. To join this list, send an e-mail to majordomo@ aamcinfo.aamc.org. Type the words "subscribe to MSAR_Clipboard" in the body, not the subject, of the message; you will be notified upon receipt

- AAMC's annual *Women in U.S. Academic Medicine Statistics* (Bickel, Croft, & Marshall, 1998) can be accessed at Website www.aamc.org/about/progemph/ wommed/stats/start.htm,

- *Enhancing the Environment for Women in Academic Medicine: Resources and Pathways* (Bickel, Croft & Marshall, 1996) is downloadable from the following AAMC Website: www.aamc.org/about/progemph/wommed/wimguide/start. htm.

American Medical Association (AMA): www.ama-assn.org; telephone: 312/ 464-5000. The AMA is a membership organization representing approximately 300,000 physicians and medical students. AMA publications of possible interest to students include the following:

- *Journal of the American Medical Association,* a monthly journal on clinical science, disease prevention and health policy issues (table of contents available on the Web)

- *American Medical News,* weekly news about professional, social, economic, and policy issues in medicine

AMA's Women in Medicine (WIM) Advisory Panel and WIM Services offer some activities in support of women in medicine (e.g., they have endorsed gender neutral language in all medical communications and also created an internal women's health office). The AMA *WIM Data Source* (available on the Website) includes statistical data on physicians by gender, age, specialty, practice characteristics, and income. Call 312/645-4392 for more information about AMA's women and minority services.

American Medical Student Association (AMSA): www.amsa.org; telephone: (800) 767-2266. AMSA is a student-governed, national organization representing approximately 30,000 medical students, premedical students, and residents across the United States. AMSA has local chapters at most medical schools and premedical chapters at over 400 universities for special community projects, educational reform efforts, and other networking activities. AMSA holds an annual meeting and offers regional workshops for students to explore medical education and health care issues with both local and national leaders; a Chapter Officers Conference helps chapter officers develop leadership skills.

A legislative affairs director (medical student) represents AMSA members on Capitol Hill, coordinates grassroots activities and educates members on health policy issues. AMSA also has various health policy fellowship and internship programs to help interested students gain the knowledge and analytical skills necessary to understand health policy and experience firsthand the legislative process. Among its many standing committees is the Women in Medicine (WIM) Committee which advocates for the interests of women in medicine and women patients, and promotes women's health education, and works to protect women's reproductive freedom. The WIM Committee offers networking opportunities through its collaboration with AMWA, as well as a listserve and newsletter.

The national office maintains a Resource Center, a variety of electronic discussion fora and an Online Residency Directory. The *New Physician Magazine,* an AMSA member benefit, covers the social, ethical and political issues facing medical education and health care.

Association of Professors of Gynecology and Obstetrics: telephone: (202) 863-2507. Women's Health competencies may be obtained from APGO, 491 12th Street, SW, Washington, DC 20024.

Women's Specialty Organizations

Although participation in mainstream organized medicine is essential to developing networks, many women have formed specialty groups within their respective disciplines. Positive results and resources have emerged, including improved networking opportunities, investigative collaborations, and formulation of policy changes adopted by the particular discipline or group.

AAMC's Women in Medicine office maintains a list of these highly diverse organizations: www.aamc.org/wim; telephone: (202) 828-0521. A few examples follow:

American Medical Women's Association (AMWA): www.amwa-doc.org; telephone: (703) 838-0500. AMWA is an independent network of more than 10,000 women physicians and medical students nationwide. It holds annual, interim, regional, and branch meetings, and offers opportunities to serve on special committees (including a Student Committee) and many member discounts. AMWA has membership chapters across the United States for local activities and projects. AMWA publishes *The Journal of the American Medical Women's Association (JAMWA)* and a variety of periodic booklets. One AMWA resource is a Gender Equity Information Line, 1-800-995-AMWA, which offers telephone advice to women physicians, residents, and students experiencing gender discrimination or sexual harassment.

Committee on Women in Science and Engineering (CWSE): www2.nas. edu/cwse. A division of the National Research Council, CWSE was founded to increase the number of women in science and engineering through activities, meetings, and research. CWSE maintains a directory (available on their Website) of professional organizations which support the education and employment of women in science and engineering.

Association for Women in Science (AWIS): www.awis.org; telephone: (202) 326-8940. AWIS is a national nonprofit organization of over 4,500 members working together to promote educational and employment opportunities for women and girls in all fields of science, mathematics, and engineering. Events at more than 50 local chapters across the country are designed to facilitate networking between women scientists at all levels and in all career paths. AWIS chapters also encourage the participation of girls and women in science by sponsoring educational activities in schools and communities. AWIS publishes a variety of materials to inform girls and women about science programs and women's issues, including the bimonthly *AWIS Magazine.*

Gay and Lesbian Medical Association (GLMA): www.glma.org; telephone: (415) 255-4547. GLMA represents over 1,900 physician and medical student members who seek to address homophobia within the medical profession by promoting the best health care for lesbian, gay, bisexual, transgendered, and HIV-positive people. In addition to meetings and special projects, GLMA publishes the *Journal of the Gay and Lesbian Medical Association,* a peer-reviewed, multidisciplinary journal dedicated to lesbian and gay health. GLMA holds an annual Women in Medicine conference for its membership to discuss current lesbian health issues.

The Association of Women Surgeons (AWS): www.womensurgeons.org; telephone: (630) 655-0392. AWS publishes a *Pocket Mentor,* a survival guide for new surgeons which fits nicely into a "white coat" pocket. This resource includes suggestions for getting organized, understanding politics, and finding mentors.

American Association for Women Radiologists (AAWR): www.aawr.org; telephone: (703) 648-8939.

Additional Internet Resources

- *Department of Health and Human Services (DHHS) www.dhhs.gov:* Agencies, news and public affairs, research, policy and administration, health information. For more information about DHHS U.S. Public Health Service Office on Women's Health and the designated Centers of Excellence in Women's Health (COE), contact ttp://www.4women.org/owh/aboutowh.htm; telephone: 1-800/994-WOMAN.

- *Food and Drug Administration (FDA) www.fda.gov:* Consumer and industry information, education, state and local officials

- *La Leche League International www.lalecheleague.org; telephone: (847) 519-7730*

- *National Library of Medicine (NLM) www.nlm.nih.gov:* Free medical literature searches, health information resources, research programs, grants

- *National Science Foundation (NSF) www.nsf.gov:* Education projects, grants and awards, fellowship support

- *National Institutes of Health (NIH) www.nih.gov:* Institutes and offices, news and information, health information, scientific opportunities, research training, grants

- *National Women's Health Information Center www.4woman.org/owh/index.htm:* Health information, references, current events, women's programs

References

American Academy of Pediatrics. (1997). Policy statement: Breastfeeding and the use of human milk. *Pediatrics, 100,*(6), 1035-1039.

American Medical Association. (1996). Women in medicine data source: A comparison of men and women physicians by specialty. In *Physician characteristics and distribution in the U.S.* Chicago: Author.

Association of Professors of Gynecology and Obstetrics. (1996). *Essential learning objectives in women's health.* Washington, DC: Author.

Andrew, L. (1996). Mentoring relationships: An evolving model. *Emergency Physician Interim Communique, 8,* 6-8.

Andrew, L. B., & Bickel, J. (1998). Gender issues in physician career development. *Career Planning and Adult Development Journal, 14,* 104-123.

Baker, L. (1996). Differences in earnings between male and female physicians. *New England Journal of Medicine, 334,* 960-964.

Baldwin, E. N., & Friedman, K. A. (1998). *A current summary of breastfeeding legislation in the U.S.* N. Miami Beach, FL: La Leche League International.

Barreca, R. (1991). *They used to call me snow white . . . but I drifted: Women's strategic use of humor.* New York: Penguin Books.

Bateson, M. C. (1990). *Composing a life.* New York: Penguin Books.

Beiser, C., & Roberts, J. (1994). Medical marriages: Opportunities and challenges of the '90s. *British Medical Journal, 309,* 1673.

Benokraitis, J. V. (Ed.). (1997). *Subtle sexism: Current practices and prospects for change.* Thousand Oaks, CA: Sage.

Bergen, M. R., Guarino, C. M., & Jacobs, C. D. (1996). A climate survey for medical students: A means to access change. *Evaluation & the Health Professions, 19,* 30-47.

Bertakis, K. D., Helms, L. J., Callahan, E. J., Azari, R., & Robinson, J. A. (1995). The influence of gender on physician practice style. *Medical Care, 33,* 407-416.

Bickel, J. (1989). Maternity leave policies for residents: An overview of issues and problems. *Academic Medicine, 64,* 498-501.

Bickel, J. (1994). Special needs and affinities of women medical students. In E. S. More & M. A. Milligan (Eds.), *The Empathic Practitioner: Empathy, Gender and Medicine* (pp. 237-250). New Brunswick, NJ: Rutgers University Press.

Bickel, J. (Ed.). (1996). Proceedings of the AAMC conference on students' and residents' ethical and professional development. *Academic Medicine, 71,* 622-642.

Bickel, J. (1997). Gender stereotypes and misconceptions: Unresolved issues in physicians' professional development. *Journal of the American Medical Association, 277,* 1405-1406.

Bickel, J., Croft, K., & Marshall, R. (1996). *Enhancing the environment for women in academic medicine: Resources and pathways.* Washington, DC: Association of American Medical Colleges.

Bickel, J., Croft, K., & Marshall, R. (1998). *Women in U.S. academic medicine statistics, 1998.* Washington, DC: Association of American Medical Colleges.

Bickel, J., & Ruffin, A. (1994). Gender-associated differences in matriculating and graduating medical students. *Academic Medicine, 70,* 552-559.

Blackstock, D. (1996). A black woman in medicine. In D. Wear (Ed.), *Women in medical education: An anthology of experience* (pp. 75-80). Albany, NY: State University of New York Press.

Bower, D., Diehr, S., Morzinski, J., & Simpson, D. E. (1998). Support-challenge-vision: A model for faculty mentoring. *Medical Teacher, 20,* 595-597.

Brooks, F. (1998). Women in general practice: Responding to the sexual division of labour? *Social Science and Medicine, 47,* 181-193.

Brotherton, S. E., & LeBailly, S. A. (1992). The effect of family on the work lives of married physicians. *Journal of the American Medical Women's Association, 48,* 322-326.

Buchanan, C. (1996). *Choosing to lead: Women and the crisis of American values.* Boston: Beacon.

Bulger, R. (1998). *The quest for mercy: The forgotten ingredient in health care reform.* Charlottesville, VA: Carden Jennings.

Calkins, E. V., Willoughby, T. L., & Arnold. L. M. (1992). Women medical students' ratings of the required surgery clerkship: Implications for career choice. *Journal of the American Medical Women's Association, 47,* 58-60.

Candib, L. (1995). *Medicine and the family: A feminist perspective.* New York: Basic Books.

Cantor, D. & Bernay, T. (1991). *Women in power: The secrets of leadership.* New York: Houghton Mifflin.

Caplan, P. (1993). *Lifting a ton of feathers: A woman's guide to surviving the academic world.* Buffalo, NY: University of Toronto Press.

Carlson, B. (1999). The new health care team. *Physician Executive, 25,* 67-75.

Carr, P., Ash, A. S., Friedman, R. H., Scaramucci, A., Barnett, R. C., Szalacha, L., Palepu, A., & Moskowitz, M. A. (1998). The relation of family responsibilities and sex to the productivity and career satisfaction of medical faculty. *Annals of Internal Medicine, 129,* 532-538.

Carr, P., Friedman, R. H., Moskowitz, M. A., & Kazis, L. E. (1993). Comparing the status of women and men in academic medicine. *Annals of Internal Medicine, 119,* 908-913.

Chow, K. (1997). Report: Maternal health and leave policies during medical training. *Journal of the American Medical Association, 277,*(9), 768-769.

Cohen, J. J. (1999). Lining up with students against abuse. *Academic Medicine, 74,* 45.

Conley, F. (1998). *Walking out on the boys.* New York: Farrar, Strauss & Giroux.

Cook, D. J., Griffith, L. E., Cohen, M., Guyatt, G. H., & O'Brien, B. (1995). Discrimination and abuse experienced by general internists in Canada. *Journal of General Internal Medicine, 10,* 565-572.

Coontz, S. (1992). *The way we never were: American families and the nostalgia trap.* New York: Basic Books.

Council on Graduate Medical Education. (1995). *Fifth report: Women and medicine.* Washington, DC: Department of Health and Human Services.

Crandall, S. J. S., Volk, R. J., & Loemker, V. (1993). Medical students' attitudes toward providing care for the underserved: Are we training socially responsible physicians? *Journal of the American Medical Association, 269,* 2519-2523.

Decade of the Executive Woman, 1982-1992. (1993). New York: Catalyst.

Doherty, W. J., & Bruge, S. K. (1989). Divorce among physicians with other occupational groups. *Journal of the American Medical Association, 261,* 2374-2377.

Donaldson, M., & Donaldson, M. (1996). *Negotiating for dummies*. Foster City, CA:IDG Books.

Dresler, C. M., Padgett D. L., MacKinnon, S. E., & Patterson, G. A. (1996). Experiences of women in cardiothoracic surgery: A gender comparison. *Archives of Surgery, 13,* 1128-1134.

Ephgrave, K. (1995). Women surgeons and the "mommy track." *Association of Women Surgeons Newsletter, 7,* 3-4.

Epps, R. P., & Stewart, S. C. (1995). *The women's complete healthbook.* New York: Delacorte.

Falik, M., & Scott-Collins, K. S. (Eds.). (1996). *Women's health: The commonwealth fund survey.* Baltimore: Johns Hopkins University Press.

Feldman, D. S., Novack, D. H., & Gracely, E. (1998). Effects of managed care on physician-patient relationships, quality of care, and the ethical practice of medicine. *Archives of Internal Medicine, 158,* 1626-1632.

Fields, S., & Toffler, W. (1993). Hopes and concerns of a first-year medical school class. *Medical Education, 27,* 124-129.

Fisher, R., & Ury, W. (1981). *Getting to yes: Negotiating agreement without giving in.* New York: Penguin.

Fiske, S. (1993). Controlling other people: The impact of power on stereotyping. *American Psychologist, 48,* 621-628.

Fletcher, R., & Fletcher, S. (1993). Here come the couples. *Annals of Internal Medicine, 119,* 628-630.

Flower, J. (1999). Living in the question. *Physician Executive, 25,* 76-78.

Fox, Y. (1998). How to negotiate a contract. *Resident and Staff Physician, 44,* 79-82.

Frank, E., Brogan, D., & Schiffman, M. (1998). Prevalence and correlates of harassment among U.S. women physicians. *Archives of Internal Medicine, 158,* 352-358.

Frank, E., Brogan, D. J., Mokdad, A. H., Simoes, E. J., Kahn, H. S., & Greenberg, R. S. (1998). Health-related behaviors of women physicians vs other women in the United States. *Archives of Internal Medicine, 158,* 342-348.

Frank, E., Rothenberg, R., Brown, W. V., & Maibach, H. (1997). Basic demographic and professional characteristics of U.S. women physicians. *Western Journal of Medicine, 166,*(3), 179-184.

Fried, L., Francomano, C. A., MacDonald, S. M., Wagner, E. M., Stokes, E. J., Carbone, K. M., Bias, W. B., Newman, M. M., & Stobo, J. D. (1996). Career development for women in academic medicine: Multiple interventions in one department of medicine. *Journal of the American Medical Association, 276,* 898-905.

Geis, F. & Butler, D. (1990). Nonverbal affect responses to male and female leaders: Implications for leadership evaluations. *Journal of Personality and Social Psychology, 58,* 48-59.

Gilligan, C. (1990). Teaching Shakespeare's sister. In C. Gilligan, N. Lyons, & T. Hamner (Eds.), *Making connections: The related worlds of adolescent girls at Emma Willard School* (pp. 6-27). Cambridge, MA: Harvard University Press.

Gjerdingen, D., Chaloner, K. M., & Vanderscoff, J. A. (1995). Family practice residents' maternity leave experiences and benefits. *Family Medicine, 27,* 512-518.

Grady-Weliky, T., Kettyle, C., & Hundert, E. (in press). New light on needs in the mentor-mentee relationship. In D. Wear & J. Bickel (Eds.), *Professional development in medical education: Curricular, clinical, and community implications.* Iowa City: University of Iowa Press.

Haapanen, K., Ellsbury, K. E., Schaad, D. C. (1996). Gender differences in the perceptions of mentorship among first- and second-year medical students. *Academic Medicine, 71,* 794.

Haas, J. (1998). The cost of being a woman. *New England Journal of Medicine, 338,* 1694-1695.

Hafferty, F. J. (1991). *Into the valley: Death and the socialization of medical students.* New Haven, CT: Yale University Press.

Haid, R. L. (1998). Preface to special issue: The changing landscape of career development in medicine. *Career Planning and Adult Development Journal, 14,* 5-6.

Hall, J., Irish, J., Roter, D., Ehrlich, C., & Miller, L. (1994). Gender in medical encounters: An analysis of physician and patient communication in a primary setting. *Health Psychology, 13,* 384-392.

Hall, L. (1992). *Negotiation: Strategies for mutual gain.* Newbury Park, CA: Sage.

Harris, D. L., Osborn, L. M., Schuman, K. L., Reading, J. C., Prather, M. B., & Politzer, R. M. (1990). Implications of pregnancy for residents and their training programs. *Journal of the American Medical Women's Association, 45,* 127-131.

Healy, B. (1995). *A new prescription for women's health: Getting the best medical care in a man's world.* New York: Penguin.

Heim, P. (1993). *Hardball for women: Winning at the game of business.* New York: Penguin.

Heinig, S. J., Quon, A. S., Meyer, R. E., & Korn, D. (1999). The changing landscape for clinical research. *Academic Medicine, 74,* 726-745.

Hickey, M., & Salmans, S. (1994). *The working mother's guilt guide: Whatever you're doing, it isn't enough.* New York: Penguin Books.

Hippensteele, S., & Pearson, T. C. (1999). Responding effectively to sexual harassment: Victim advocacy, early intervention, and problem-solving. *Change, 31,* 48-53.

Hostler, S., & Gressard, R. (1993). Perceptions of gender fairness of the medical education environment. *Journal of the American Medical Women's Association, 48,* 51-54.

Hunt, K., & Allandale, E. (1999). Relocating gender and morbidity: Examining men's and women's health in contemporary western societies. *Social Science and Medicine, 48,* 1-5.

Iserson, K. (1996). *Getting into a residency: A guide for medical students.* Tucson, AZ: Galen.

James, J. (1997). Thinking in the future tense. *Healthcare Forum Journal, 40,*(1), 26-31.

Jamieson, K. (1995). *Beyond the double bind: Women and leadership.* New York: Oxford University Press.

Jeruchim, J., & Shapiro, P. (1992). *Women, mentors, and success.* New York: Ballantine Books.

Jonassen, J. A., Pugnaire, M. P., Mazor, K., Regan, M. B., Jacobson, E. W., Gammon, W., Doepel, D. G., & Cohen, A. J. (1999). The effect of a domestic violence interclerkship on the knowledge, attitudes, and skills of third-year medical students. *Academic Medicine, 74,* 821-828.

Justice, A., & Mulrow, C. (1995). When the patient abuses the physician. *Journal of General Internal Medicine, 10,* 588-589.

Kaltreider, N. (Ed.). (1997). *Dilemmas of a double life: Women balancing careers and relationships.* Northvale, NJ: Jason Aronson.

Kaplan, S. H., Sullivan, L. M., Dukes, K. A., Phillips, C. F., Kelch, R. P., & Schaller, J. G. (1996). Sex differences in academic advancement: Results of a national study of pediatricians. *New England Journal of Medicine, 335,* 1282-1289.

Kassebaum, D. G., & Cutler, E. R. (1998). On the culture of student abuse in medical school. *Academic Medicine, 73,* 1149-1158.

Kiely Law, J. (1997). Pulse: Starting a family in medical school. *Journal of the American Medical Association, 277,*(9), 767.

King, J. A. (1995). *The smart woman's guide to interviewing and salary negotiation* (2nd ed.). Franklin Lakes, NJ: Career Press.

Klebanoff, M. A., Shiono, P. H., & Rhoads, G. G. (1990). Outcomes of pregnancy in a national sample of resident physicians. *New England Journal of Medicine, 323,* 1040-1045.

Klebanoff, M. A., Shiono, P. H., & Rhoads, G. G. (1991). Spontaneous and induced abortion among resident physicians. *Journal of the American Medical Association, 265,* 2821-2825.

Komaromy, M., Bindman, A. B., Haber, R. J., & Sande, M. A. (1993). Sexual harassment in medical training. *New England Journal of Medicine, 328,* 322-326.

Kritek, P. (1996). *Negotiating at an uneven table: A practical approach to dealing with difference and diversity.* San Francisco: Jossey Bass.

Krueger, P. M. (1998). Do women medical students outperform men in obstetrics and gynecology? *Academic Medicine, 73,* 101-102.

Kwolek, D. S., Griffith, C. H., & Blue, A. V. (1999). Using clinical skills workshops to teach complex assessment skill in women's health. *Teaching and Learning in Medicine, 11,* 105-109.

Lane, A. J. (1998). Consensual relations in the academy: Gender, power, and sexuality. *Academe, 84,* 24-31.

Leider, R. J. (1995). *Repacking your bags: Lighten your load for the rest of your life.* San Francisco: Berrett-Koehler.

Lent, B., & Bishop, J. (1998). Sense and sensitivity: Developing a gender issues perspective in medical education [abstract]. *Journal of Women's Health, 7,*(3).

Levinson, W., Tolle, S. W., & Lewis, C. (1989). Women in academic medicine: Combining career and family. *New England Journal of Medicine, 321,* 1511-1517.

Levinson, W. (1989). Position paper: Parental leave for residents. *Annals of Internal Medicine, 111,* 1035-1038.

Limacher, M. C., Zaher, C. A., Walsh, M. N., Wolf, W. J., Douglas, P. S., Schwartz, J. B., Wright, J. S., & Bodycombe, D. P. (1998). The ACC professional life survey: Career decisions of women and men in cardiology. *Journal of the American College of Cardiology, 32,* 827-835.

Linney, B. (1999). Medical marriages. *Physician Executive, 25,* 81-83.

Little, M. O. (1996). Why a feminist approach to bioethics? *Kennedy Institute of Ethics Journal, 6,* 1-18.

Lovejoy, E. P. (1957). *Women doctors of the world.* New York: Macmillan.

Luchetti, C. (1998). *Medicine women: The story of early-American women doctors.* New York: Crown.

Lurie, N., Slater, J., McGovern, P., Ekstrum, J., Quam, L., & Margolis, K.. 1993. Preventive care for women: Does the sex of the physician matter? *New England Journal of Medicine, 329,* 478-482.

Mangus, R. S., Hawkins, C. E., & Miller, J. J. (1998). Prevalence of harassment and discrimination among 1996 medical school graduates: A survey of eight U.S. schools. *Journal of the American Medical Association, 280,* 851-853.

Marshall, E. (1997). Women's health research: A 5-year initiative slowly takes shape. *Science, 278,* 1558.

Mendelsohn, K. D., Nieman, L. Z., Isaacs, K., Lee, S., & Levison, S. P. (1994). Sex and gender bias in anatomy and physical diagnosis text illustrations. *Journal of the American Medical Association, 272,* 1267-1270.

Miles, S., & Parker, K. (1997). Men, women, and health insurance. *New England Journal of Medicine, 336,* 218-220.

Miles, S., & August, A. (1990). Courts, gender, and the right to die. *Law, Medicine & Health Care, 18,* 85-95.

Miller, R. S., Dunn, M. R., Richter, T. H., & Whitcomb, M. E. (1998). Employment-seeking experiences of resident physicians completing training during 1996. *Journal of the American Medical Association, 280,* 777-783.

Mindell, P. A. (1995). *A woman's guide to the language of success: Communicating with confidence and power.* Englewood Cliffs, NJ: Prentice Hall.

Molidor, J. B., & Barber, K.R. (1998). I can't believe you asked that! *Academic Medicine, 73,* 731-732.

Morantz-Sanchez, R. (1985). *Sympathy & science: Women physicians in American medicine.* New York: Oxford University Press.

Morantz-Sanchez, R. (1994). The gendering of empathic expertise: How women physicians became more empathic than men. In E. More & M. Milligan (Eds.), *The empathic practitioner: Empathy, gender and medicine* (pp. 40-58). New Brunswick, NJ: Rutgers University Press.

Moscarello, R., Katalin, J. M., & Rossi, M. (1996). Impact of faculty education on the incidence of sexual harassment experienced by Canadian medical students. *Journal of Women's Health, 5,* 231-237.

Mutha, S., Takayama, J. I., & O'Neil, E. H. (1997). Insights into medical students' career choices based on third- and fourth-year students' focus-group discussions. *Academic Medicine, 72,* 635-640.

National Academy of Women's Health in Medical Education. (1996). Definition of women's health. In G. D. Donoghue (Ed.)., *Women's health in the curriculum: A resource guide for faculty* (pp. 3-4). MCP-Philadelphia: Hahnemann School of Medicine/Author.

Nelson, M., Nicolete, J., & Johnson, K. (1997). Integration or evolution: Women's health as a model for interdisciplinary change in medical education. *Academic Medicine, 72,* 737-740.

Neumayer, L., Levinson, W., & Putnam, C. (1995). Mentors for women in surgery and their effect on career advancement. *Current Surgery, 52,* 163-166.

Nora, L. M., Daugherty, S. R., Hersh, K., Schmidt, J., & Goodman, L. J. (1993). What do medical students mean when they say "sexual harassment?" *Academic Medicine, 68,*(Suppl. 10), S49-51.

Notman, M. T., Salt, P., & Nadelson, C. C. (1984). Stress and adaptation in medical students: Who is the most vulnerable? *Comprehensive Psychiatry, 25,* 355-356.

Osborn, E. H. S., Ernster, V. L., & Martin, J. B. (1992). Women's attitudes toward careers in academic medicine at the University of California, San Francisco. *Academic Medicine, 67,* 59-62.

Osborn, L. M., Harris, D. L., Reading, J. C., & Prather, M. B. (1990). Outcome of pregnancies experience during residency. *The Journal of Family Practice, 31,* 616-622.

Palepu, A., Friedman, R. H., Barnett, R. C., Carr, P. L., Ash, A. S., Moskowitz, M. A., & Szalacha, L. (1996). Medical faculty with mentors are more satisfied. *Journal of General Internal Medicine, 11,*(Suppl.), 107.

Pearson, T. (1998). Physician employees: The new social contract in health care. *Career Planning and Adult Development Journal, 14,* 43-58.

Philibert, I., & Bickel, J. (1995). Maternity and parental leave policies at COTH hospitals: An update. *Academic Medicine, 70,* 1056-1058.

Phillips, S., & Schneider, M. (1993). Sexual harassment of female doctors by patients. *New England Journal of Medicine, 329,* 1936-1939.

President and Fellows of Harvard College. (1998). *Family Resource Handbook.* Boston: Harvard Medical Center Office of Work and Family & Harvard University Office of Work and Family.

Ragins, B. R., & Cotton, J. (1993). Gender and willingness to mentor in organizations. *Journal of Management, 19,* 97-111.

Rhode, D. (1997). *Speaking of sex: The denial of gender inequality.* Cambridge, MA: Harvard University Press.

Rollman, B. L., Mead, L. A., Wang, N. Y., & Klag, M. J. (1997). Occasional notes: Medical specialty and the incidence of divorce. *New England Journal of Medicine, 336,*(11), 800-803.

Rosenfield, N. (1998). *Child care: A combined experience from the American Association of Women Radiologists.* Reston, VA: AAWR.

Roth Walsh, M. (1977). *Doctors wanted: No women need apply, sexual barriers in the medical profession, 1835-1975.* New Haven, CT: Yale University Press.

Rothman, E. L. (1999). *White coat: Becoming a doctor at Harvard Medical School.* Boston: William Morrow.

Sandler, B., & Shoop, R. (1997). *Sexual harassment on campus: A guide for administrators, faculty and students.* Boston: Allyn & Bacon.

Sandler, B., Silverberg, L., & Hall, R. (1996). *The chilly classroom climate: A guide to improve the education of women.* Washington, DC: National Association of Women in Education.

Schulman, K.A., & Berlin, J.A. (1999). The effect of race and sex on physicians' recommendations for cardiac catheterization. *New England Journal of Medicine, 340,* 618-625.

Schapiro, N. (1993). *Negotiating for your life: New success strategies for women.* New York: Henry Holt.

Schwartz, F. N., Schifter, M. H., & Gillotti, S. S. (1972). *How to go to work when your husband is against it, your children aren't old enough, and there's nothing you can do anyhow.* New York: Catalyst.

Secundy, M. G. (1996). Life as sheep in the cow's pasture. In D. Wear (Ed.), *Women in medical education: An anthology of experience* (p. 121). Albany, NY: State University of New York Press.

Sells, J., & Sells, C. (1989). Pediatrician and parent: A challenge for female physicians. *Pediatrics, 84,* 355-361.

Seltzer, V., & Pearse, W. (1995). *Women's primary health care: Office practice and procedures.* New York: McGraw-Hill.

Senge, P., Kleiner, A., Roberts, C., Ross, R., & Smith, B. (1999). *A fifth discipline resource. The dance of change: The challenges to sustaining momentum in learning organizations.* New York: Doubleday.

Shervington, D. O., Bland, I. J., & Myers, A. (1996). Ethnicity, gender identity, stress, and coping among female African-American medical students. *Journal of the American Medical Women's Association, 51,* 153-154.

Siders, C. T., & Aschenbrener, C. A. (1999). Conflict management checklist: A diagnostic tool for assessing conflict in organizations. *Physician Executive, 25,* 32-37.

Sonnert, G., & Holton, G. (1995). *Who succeeds in science? The gender dimension.* New Brunswick, NJ: Rutgers University Press.

Sotile, W. M., & Sotile, M. O. (1998). *Supercouple syndrome: How overworked couples can beat stress together.* New York: John Wiley.

St. James, D. (1996). *Writing and speaking for excellence: A guide for physicians.* Boston: Jones & Bartlett.

Tannen, D. (1995). *Talking from 9 to 5: Language, sex & power.* New York: Avon.

Tesch, B. J., Wood, H. M., Helwig, A. L., & Nattinger, A. B. (1995). Promotion of women physicians: Glass ceiling or sticky floor? *Journal of the American Medical Association, 273,* 1022-1025.

Tesch, B. J., Osborne, J., Simpson, D. E., Murray, S. F., & Spiro, J. (1992). Women physicians in dual-physician relationships compared with those in other dual-career relationships. *Academic Medicine, 67,* 542-544.

Thomas, K. W. (1992). Conflict and conflict management. *Journal of Organizational Behavior, 13,* 265-274.

Tidball, M. E., Smith, D. G., Tidball, C. S., & Wolf-Wendell, L. E. (1998). *Taking women seriously: Lessons & legacies for educating the majority.* Washington, DC: Oryx Press/American Council on Education.

Tobin J. N., Wassertheil-Smoller, S., Wexler, J. P., Steingart, R. M., Budner, N., Lense, L., & Wachpress, J. (1987). Sex bias in considering coronary bypass surgery. *Annals of Internal Medicine, 107,* 19-25.

Tom, S. C. (1997). Opening the doors to medical education: From the Victorian era to the present. *Initiative, 58,*(2), 23-37.

Tronto, J. (1995). Sexism. In W. Reich (Ed.)., *Encyclopedia of bioethics.* New York: Simon & Schuster.

Turk, M. (1997, April). In love and medicine. *The New Physician,* pp. 21-24.

Valian, V. (1998). *Why so slow: The advancement of women.* Cambridge: MIT Press.

vanIneveld, C. H., Cook, D. J., Kane, S. L., & King, D. (1996). Discrimination and abuse in internal medicine residency. *Journal of General Internal Medicine, 3,* 401-405.

Varner, K. (Ed.). (1999). *Curriculum directory.* Washington, DC: Association of American Medical Colleges.

Varner, K. (Ed.). (1999). *Medical school admission requirements.* Washington, DC: Association of American Medical Colleges.

Wallis, L. (1998). *Textbook of women's health.* Philadelphia: Lippincott-Raven.

Warde, C., Allen, W., & Gelberg, L. (1996). Physician role conflict and resulting career changes: Gender and generational differences. *Journal of General Internal Medicine, 11,* 729-735.

Weeks, D. (1992). *The eight essential steps to conflict resolution.* Los Angeles: Jeremy Tarcher.

Weisman, C .S. (1998). *Women's health care: Activist traditions and institutional change.* Baltimore: Johns Hopkins University Press.

Whitfill, J. T. (1998). Reflections on the annual meeting. *Society of General Internal Medicine Forum, 21,*(8), 2.

Wiebe, C. (1997). Parenthood and residency: The great balancing act. *American College of Physicians Observer, 17,* 6-7.

Wilke, A. J. (1999). When a resident is incapacitated. *Family Medicine, 31,* 384-386.

Wolf, W. (1998, December). *The art of self promotion.* Paper presented at AAMC Professional Development Seminar for Junior Women Faculty, Santa Fe, NM.

Xu, G. Veloski, J., & Hojat, M. (1998). Board certification: Associations with physicians' demographics and performances during medical school and residency. *Academic Medicine, 73,* 1283-1289.

Yale University School of Medicine. (1998). *Tell someone.* New Haven, CT: Author.

Author Index

Subject Index

About the Author

Janet Bickel, MA, is Associate Vice President of the Association of American Medical Colleges (AAMC), Division of Institutional Planning and Development. She has worked at the forefront of medical education for over 25 years, most recently concentrating on issues of women's professional development. She has spoken at over 60 academic medical centers on these issues and published articles on these and a broad spectrum of other areas in academic medicine, including students' and residents' ethical development. Ms. Bickel created a series of professional development seminars for potential women leaders in academic medicine which has received excellent reviews from the over 2,000 faculty who have attended. Prior to directing AAMC's Women in Medicine program, Ms. Bickel staffed AAMC's Organization of Medical Student Representatives, composed of student leaders from all U.S. medical schools; this work included writing an issue-oriented newsletter received by all 16,000 medical students in the country. Her involvement with medical education began at Brown University where she served as admissions, financial aid, and student affairs officer for the new medical school between 1972 and 1976.